THE PUMP ENERGY FOOD

The Pu
Energy

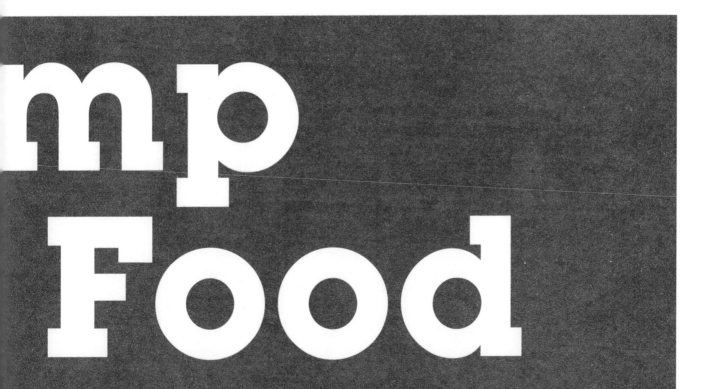

mp
Food

Steve and Elena Kapelonis
with Mary Goodbody

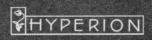 HYPERION

NEW YORK

The ideas, suggestions, and procedures in this book do not replace the medical advice of a trained medical professional. You should consult with your physician before adopting the suggestions in this book, especially if you have any preexisting medical or psychological conditions, or if you are currently taking medicine. Following these dietary suggestions may impact the effect of certain types of medication. Any changes in your dosage should be made only in cooperation with your prescribing physician.

Pregnant women are advised that special precautions may pertain to any nutritional program they undertake. If you are pregnant, talk to your doctor before undertaking the programs recommended in this book.

The author and publisher disclaim any liability directly or indirectly from the use of the material in this book by any person.

Nutritional Analysis supplied by Esha Research Inc. and the Food Processor SQL, Salem Oregon.

ISBN 1-4013-0744-2

Hyperion books are available for special promotions and premiums. For details contact Michael Rentas, Manager, Inventory and Premium Sales, Hyperion, 77 West 66th Street, 11th floor,
New York, New York 10023, or call 212-456-0133.

Designed by Doug Riccardi

FIRST EDITION

10 9 8 7 6 5 4 3 2

This book is dedicated to each and every one of us who tries to make the world a better place by becoming a better person.

Acknowledgments

Thank you to our families, employees, customers, editors, and agent.
Thank you, Steven Ratushewitz, for your everlasting and inspirational memories.

Contents

Foreword **xi**

Introduction **xiii**

1: Join Us at the Pump **3**

2: Appetizers **13**

3: Soups and Sandwiches **23**

4: Salads **37**

5: Fish and Seafood **63**

6: Lean Meat and Poultry **75**

7: Vegetarian Main Courses **97**

8: Pizza and Burgers **109**

9: **Vegetable Sides 123**

10: **Pump Shakes and Juices 141**

11: **Dressings and Sauces 167**

12: **Desserts 177**

13: **Eggs and Pancakes 189**

14: **Snacks 205**

15: **Supercharged Plates 215**

16: **The Pump Energy Two-Week Meal Plans 229**

Index 246

Foreword

WE MAKE POOR FOOD CHOICES. As a nation we are infatuated with fast food. We take great care planning vacations, choosing which automobile to purchase or lease, but pay little attention to what we put in our mouths to nourish our bodies. The future of medicine will focus more on nutrition. The suppliers and providers of our healthy food are the true pharmacists, dispensing "medicine" in the form of healthy food.

According to the CDC National Center for Health Statistics, nearly two out of three (64.5 percent) adults in the United States are overweight or obese. The percentage of U.S. adults classified as obese doubled between 1980 and 2003, from 15 percent to 31 percent. Current data suggest that 20 percent of U.S. children are overweight (*American Journal of Clinical Nutrition,* vol. 73, no. 2, 158–171). Obesity continues to increase in children and adolescents, and annual obesity-related hospital costs in six- to seventeen-year-olds have reached $127 million per year. Overweight children and adolescents are now being diagnosed with impaired glucose tolerance and type 2 diabetes, and they show early signs of the insulin resistance syndrome and cardiovascular risk. Several risk factors have been identified as contributors to the development of type 2 diabetes and cardiovascular risk in youth. These factors include increased body fat and abdominal fat, insulin resistance, and onset of puberty.

Each year more American children are killed by obesity than by gun violence. Obesity is a greater trigger for health problems and increased health spending than smoking or drinking. Individuals who are obese have 30 percent to 50 percent more chronic medical problems than those who smoke or drink heavily. The effects of obesity are similar to twenty years of aging. Forty percent of U.S. adults get no leisure-time physical activity; only 14 percent meet the standard of brisk walking for 30 minutes per day, five times per week.

Overweight and obese individuals are at increased risk for diabetes; heart disease; hypertension; musculoskeletal conditions; stroke; endometrial, breast, prostate, and colon cancers; poor female reproductive health; and depression, among other conditions. Obesity is associated with 39 million lost workdays; 239 million restricted activity days; 90 million sick days; along with 63 million physician visits.

The power to control this apparent epidemic of obesity rests in the hands of all people. We have the power to change these statistics with what we put into our mouths. Poor food choices are the reason for the majority of health concerns and diseases in the human population. We need to focus on healthier eating. A whole foods diet is the easiest way to prevent obesity and numerous illnesses.

A strong foundation is required when building a home. Our bodies need to follow the same premise. A diet composed of whole grains, legumes, fresh fruits and vegetables, low-fat dairy, eggs and lean protein from poultry, lean beef, and fish builds a healthy body.

I had the pleasure of meeting Steve and Elena four years ago. We share the same vision, but approach it from two different perspectives that meet in the middle. As a clinical nutritionist, I address the health concerns of my patients with recommendations of nutritional protocols specific to them, always maintaining the foundation of a healthy diet based upon whole foods. Steve and Elena are providers of a very important service. They offer the public healthy food that builds healthy bodies, using whole foods and pure, natural ingredients. Not one item on the menu at the Pump is unhealthy. I can't apply that statement to any other restaurant. What I respect about Steve and Elena is that their commitment to providing nourishing food to the public is genuine. They share my passion for nutrition. They feed their beautiful children the same healthy food that they work so hard to provide to the public. Steve and Elena test every recipe over and over again before it leaves their kitchen and enters the Pump. They provide educational materials as handouts for the public in their restaurant. The walls are adorned with articles on nutrition and pictures of famous people, signed with praise to the Pump.

I've been eating at the Pump for the past four years, and recommend it to every patient I see in my clinical practice. I'm honored that Steve and Elena asked me to write the foreword to this book. After reviewing it, I was amazed at the wonderful recipes and quite honestly can't wait to see them reach the public. I urge everyone interested in their health and the health of their loved ones to read this book, start using the recipes as a guide to planning healthy meals, and eat food by the Pump!

—DR. ROBERT PASTORE, New York City

Introduction

EVERY DAY, THOUSANDS OF PEOPLE eat at one of our Pump Energy Food restaurants on New York's Manhattan Island. They stop in for breakfast on the way to work, buy lunch to eat at their desks or in a nearby park, and come by at the end of the day to buy supper.

Yes, the food is fresh and carefully prepared, but as we, the restaurant's two owners, hear time and again, our customers eat at the Pump because our food makes them *feel* great. It's as simple as that. As we see it, customers prefer good, wholesome food that never leaves them feeling groggy or stuffed, but, on the other hand, never leaves them feeling deprived. When you eat the Pump way, you feel fantastic.

We wrote this book because our regular customers look better than people who frequent other restaurants. In New York City, the Pump has become a lifestyle, a feeling. It's about eating the right food at the right time so that you have all the energy you need to do everything you want to do, and to do it exactly how you want to do it.

People in a healthy state of mind love Pump food. When they visit one of our restaurants, they find "food that tastes great and makes you feel and look great." Now we want to show you how to make this food at home.

We opened our first restaurant in 1997, calling it a physical fitness restaurant. This designation alone immediately set us apart from other casual eateries. We chose this tagline because we had seen firsthand how enthusiastic people were about the food Steve was preparing at juice bars in two Manhattan gyms.

We believed it was time to take the food outside the gym.

On opening day, the line of customers went out the door. On the second day, the lines were just as long—and we weren't giving away any more free samples! To this day, we recognize many faces from those early weeks.

Our philosophy is simple: Eat the right food in the right combinations and you will stay fit and healthy. Make this a lifelong commitment, and you will have all the energy you need to sail through your days with more than enough energy. What could be better?

We are not advocating a weight-loss diet, although a lot of our customers lose weight. For every customer who wants to shed pounds, we have just as many who want to build muscle. They eat our food for the energy they need to pump iron at the gym, run on the track, or finish a long day of work, which means our food is anything but skimpy.

We wrote this book to help everyone feel better and stay fit, regardless of their level of fitness, weight, and muscle mass. We don't have strict rules and complicated guidelines, but we do have strong beliefs.

First and foremost, eat the right foods. Make sure it's whole food, not processed foods. Begin the day with protein and complex carbohydrates (we don't subscribe to the idea that *all* carbs are the enemy!). Eat lots of vegetables and some fruit. Limit carbs as the day goes by so that by suppertime you are eating primarily protein and vegetables. And fat? Fat is important. Eat small amounts of good fats, such as olive and sesame oil, nuts, and avocados.

That's it. Nothing to it. Welcome to the Pump lifestyle.

THE PUMP ENERGY FOOD

01.
Join Us at the Pump

WHEN YOU DECIDE TO EAT AND LIVE the Pump way, you will feel and look better. You will have dynamic energy and all the motivation you need to reach your personal fitness goals. You don't have to be an athlete to benefit from the Pump. Many of our customers are professional dancers, artists, and actors; some of them have high-stress desk jobs that require them to be inactive for most of the day. Our customers all share one thing: They are interested in staying fit and rely on us to fuel their bodies and their minds. Our customers tell us that our food works for them. It's why we wrote this book.

This book is packed with great recipes that address managing your lifestyle so that you get optimal enjoyment from life. Without question, if you want to lose weight, our recipes will help. Turn to page 230 for a comprehensive two-week meal plan to help you shed pounds. On the other hand, if you want to build muscle, turn to page 238 for an equally comprehensive meal plan to help you bulk up.

But this book is not just another diet and health book. At the restaurant, our menu is designed for athletes and other active people, yet is tasty and familiar enough for the everyday home cook to incorporate into daily meals. Nothing about our food is weird. We cook at home every night for our own two small daughters, so we know firsthand what it means to prepare family meals.

Sure, we eat some tofu (which fewer and fewer Americans classify as weird), but mainly we eat chicken, fish, beef, and lamb, just like everybody else. We understand the needs of vegetarians, too, and so have included a number of excellent vegetarian dishes.

We don't shun brown rice, grains, sweet potatoes, or fruit, as do many of the low-carbohydrate diets on the market. We couldn't get through a day without these foods. We have recipes for pizzas and burgers, too, and admit freely to our love of healthful sweets (try our apple pie!).

We always tell people that the best way to eat healthfully is to eat the *right* foods in the *right* combinations.

The Right Foods

Deciding to take charge of your health and your body is the first step. Recognizing the right foods is the next. If you are what you eat, you want to be fresh, wholesome, and lean. Stop putting the wrong foods in your mouth. Replace them with the right ones, and in a matter of weeks you will start to feel better.

Protein is the key to the Pump lifestyle and should be eaten at every meal. Combined with vegetables, protein satisfies your appetite, stimulates energy, and, if you need to, helps you lose weight. When you eat enough protein and exercise regularly, you build muscle.

THE RIGHT FOODS ARE:
- fish
- chicken
- turkey
- egg whites
- lean beef and lamb
- beans (including tofu)
- vegetables
- fruits
- nuts
- olive oil, canola oil, sesame oil
- dried fruits
- brown rice
- whole wheat pita bread
- sweet potatoes
- rice cakes

We also suggest limited amounts of dairy products, which are valuable sources of calcium.

THOSE WE LIKE ARE:

- skim milk
- plain yogurt (nonfat or low-fat yogurt)
- nonfat and low-fat cheeses

The Wrong Foods

We don't like to dwell on the negative, but how could we discuss the right foods without talking about the wrong ones?

FOODS TO AVOID ARE:

- white bread
- white pasta
- white rice
- white potatoes
- fried foods
- mayonnaise
- bacon
- egg yolks
- butter and cream
- desserts containing lots of sugar and dairy fat (such as butter and cream)
- sugary beverages

While cheese is high in protein, we suggest limiting it, and when you do eat it, eat unprocessed cheese. The amount should be so small as to be no more than a garnish, which is still enough for a flavor punch. Cheese is high in calories and salt; if you eat a lot of it, you'll retain water.

This is true of eating salty foods in general. There's no need to consume as much salt as we Americans do, which is why in nearly all our recipes we make salt optional, if we use it at all. The choice to add it is yours. Eating too much sugar will only increase your desire for it. The sooner you kick the salt and sugar habits, the better.

PUMP LIFESTYLE COOKING TOOLS TO KEEP IN YOUR KITCHEN

- Steamer for vegetables
- Oven to bake and broil
- Large pan or wok
- Baking pans
- Blender
- Cooking gloves
- The right utensils
- Big salad bowls
- Small and large drainer
- Cutting board for meat
- Cutting board for vegetables
- Small and large pots
- Plastic storage containers
- Spice rack

PUMP LIFESTYLE FOOD ESSENTIALS TO KEEP IN YOUR KITCHEN

- Cucumbers
- Tomatoes
- Onions
- Cabbage
- Romaine
- Broccoli
- Spinach
- Asparagus
- String Beans
- Avocados
- Beans
- Parsley
- Dill
- Lemons
- Eggs
- Tuna
- Chicken
- Lean Meat
- Tofu
- Olive Oil
- Cooking Spray
- Sea Salt (if you use)
- Vinegar
- Brown Rice

The Pump Kitchen

When you decide to cook the Pump way, you may have to buy a few items for your kitchen. While most of our recipes are easy to make with the pots, pans, and utensils every kitchen has, some require equipment you may not have.

For instance, we call for a juice extractor for the juices in Chapter 10. In the other recipes in the same chapter, you will need a good blender. In Chapter 13, we call for an omelet pan, although you may use a small skillet instead.

Other than these, you may want to consider an electric steamer (we use one made by GE), a countertop grill (such as the George Foreman Grill), and an immersion blender for creamy soups.

Because we feel strongly that the right tools make the job far easier, we suggest you invest in an instant-read thermometer for judging the internal temperature of meat and poultry, a mortar and pestle to crush fresh herbs and spices, and a good grater (we like the Microplaner). You will need supplies of aluminum foil, waxed paper, cheesecloth, and kitchen twine, too.

The Winning Quarter

Whether you want to lose weight or recharge your body so that it operates like a well-calibrated machine, we have developed a plan we call the Winning Quarter. Many of our customers are athletes, so we named this plan after a game-winning strategy in basketball. When a team has a great quarter with a lot of scoring, they call it the winning quarter. Unless something totally unexpected happens in the remainder of the game, this high-scoring quarter is the winning one. The game is locked up.

We feel the same way about getting into the Pump. Give yourself six weeks (less than two months!) to change your life. This will be your winning quarter and you won't regret it.

Begin with a commitment. Just as you would commit to a business plan for your job, a study plan for school, or a training regimen for a sport, commit to the Pump lifestyle for six weeks. This way you will lose body fat, define your muscles, and make them come alive. When the time is up, your only challenge will be to maintain your new body, but that will be easy. By then, you will have embraced the Pump lifestyle and sustaining it won't be tough.

HERE'S WHAT YOU DO:

- Decide to eat only good foods and enough of them.
- Eat protein with every meal.
- Eat twice as many vegetables or as much salad as protein.
- Eat carbohydrates in the morning and then taper off as the day goes on.
- Eat supper at least four hours before bedtime.
- Drink plenty of water. We recommend at least 64 ounces a day, which is only one 16-ounce bottle per meal and one with a snack.
- Limit fat. When you eat fat (and some is necessary for good health), make sure it's a good fat, such as olive oil, canola oil, and sesame oil. You can eat nuts and avocados, both fat-laden foods, in moderation, too.
- Declare war on all bread (except whole wheat pita bread and other whole grain breads), white pasta, white rice, white potatoes, mayonnaise, egg yolks, processed cheeses, fried foods, creamy or cakey desserts, and sugar-filled soft drinks and bottled juices.
- Never get hungry. Eat your snacks!
- Limit or totally avoid alcohol. We enjoy a glass of wine with dinner now and then and so can't completely rule out alcohol!
- Figure out the right supplements for you.
- Commit to 40 minutes of mildly strenuous exercise daily.
- Don't cheat. This is important. Even a bite of cheesecake or a few French fries can sabotage all your good work.

Failure Is Easy, but Success Is So Much Sweeter

We've had customers tell us that the easiest way for them to stick to a healthful regimen is to eat at the Pump five, six, or more times a week. The world is full of unhealthy temptations.

We get fat or lose muscle strength for any number of reasons. First, understand why you may have slipped over the years. Second, don't blame yourself—it's so easy to do!

Our bodies and metabolism change as we get older. We get lazy about exercising and watching our diets, and many of us give up.

We move, get injured, go through a life change, or start a new job. Any of these gives us "permission" to eat the wrong foods.

Fattening foods are cheap and easy to buy. Bags of chips, soda, candy bars, ice cream cones, and fast food burgers assault us at every turn. They are packaged for munching on the go, which only makes them more dangerous.

We don't drink enough water. When we're thirsty we reach for a soda, which does very little to quench our thirst. We may think a fruit-based drink or bottled iced tea is more beneficial than soda when in fact it's full of sugar.

There's always tomorrow. Parties, social gatherings, holidays, and family celebrations are rife with tempting foods. It's hard to curb our enthusiasm.

Once you recognize these all-too-familiar traps, you can decide to put them behind you and instead embrace success.

Strategies for Success

It took years to gain weight and lose muscle tone and flexibility, so don't expect to reverse the process overnight. It's impossible to anticipate all the pitfalls you will encounter along the way, but we've put together some tips that should help.

I have restructured my entire diet to mirror that of the Pump's menu! I find I feel just as good on the weekends now as I do during the week! Love the menu, love the results, love the Pump!
—JIM BYRNE, customer

· Write down why you want to change your life. Keep it to two or three sentences and read it often. Tape it to the refrigerator or mirror. This will keep you motivated.

· Make a list of the right foods and keep it as a reference. This is particularly handy when you crave a snack!

· Avoid the wrong foods. Sounds simple, and it is. Consider them taboo, out of the question, no-nos.

· Eat fruit to curb your desire for the wrong foods. It works!

· Plan your meals the day before. Write down the foods you will eat tomorrow. This will help you stay with the plan.

· If you eat pasta or pizza, do so early in the day and then end the day with a lot of vegetables or a salad. When you eat pasta or a pizza, double the amount of veggies you normally would toss with it or top it with and forgo all or most of the cheese.

· Exercise daily. Don't miss a day; write it on your calendar.

· Don't skip meals or snacks. Getting hungry is counterproductive, and you'll just eat more than you should.

· Limit coffee and tea. These can be pick-me-ups during the day, but we suggest two cups of coffee or tea, tops.

· Avoid salty foods. These make you retain water and also can disrupt your sleep. You need enough sleep to maintain your energy level during the day.

· Eat protein bars as snacks, not as accompaniments to meals.

· Reward yourself with something: a new outfit, a night at the movies, or a hike.

· Get back on track if you slip. Although we have urged you not to take a bite of cheesecake or even a few fries, if you do, don't give up.

· Weigh yourself at least once a week. This will help ensure you stay within five pounds of your current goal weight.

· Photograph yourself once a month and take pride in the changes you see.

· Write down your feelings and food choices. Note changes in attitude and body shape. This will keep you motivated.

· Consider the diet a journey without stress, one to be savored.

Just like you, we live in the real world. We have a young family, lots of doting relatives, and good friends. We love to get together with these folks, at our place, theirs, or a restaurant. So we know what you face when you're invited to a party or a meal out. Here are some of the ways we have learned to cope in situations where too much food and too many choices tempt our resolve.

PARTY BUFFETS: Look for the primary protein (usually chicken, turkey, beef, fish, or beans), unadorned vegetables, and salads. Stay away from mashed or roasted potatoes, bread of any kind, and pasta preparations. Eat fruit or a small piece of chocolate for dessert. Stay away from creamy desserts, cookies, and cakes.

RESTAURANTS: Don't order appetizers. Ask for a small green salad instead. If you order a main course that comes with rice, pasta, or potatoes, ask to substitute salad or steamed vegetables for the carbs. Make sure the protein you order is lean chicken, beef, or fish without a heavy cream sauce.

CHINESE AND JAPANESE RESTAURANTS: At a Chinese restaurant, stick with chicken and broccoli or beef or tofu with string beans or asparagus. In other words, order a sensible protein with lots of vegetables. Eat only a little of the sauce and avoid the rice, dumplings, and noodles. Ask that your food be made without cornstarch, which reduces calories and makes the sauces thinner and lighter. At a Japanese restaurant, eat sashimi (fish without the rice) or beef, tofu, or chicken teriyaki. Ask for only half the sauce. Miso soup is a good choice, too. Hold back on the soy sauce and other dipping sauces and use only a little low-sodium soy sauce. Don't eat too much rice.

FAST FOOD RESTAURANTS: Stay away from fried foods such as French fries, onion rings, and battered chicken and fish.

Order a grilled chicken sandwich or a burger without cheese and eat only the meat and vegetables. You may need to order two sandwiches to satisfy your appetite, but that's better than eating all that bread. If the restaurant has a salad (and many do), eat it with very little dressing.

DELICATESSENS: Order meat sandwiches—pastrami, corned beef, or turkey—but ditch the bread. Use mustard to flavor the protein instead of mayonnaise. If you can, order steamed veggies with the meat or pick and choose from a salad bar.

BALL GAME, OUTDOOR FAIR, OR MOVIE THEATER: Eat the hot dogs, with or without mustard, but don't eat the bun. Drink diet soda if you can't get water. Snack on unbuttered popcorn.

Welcome to the Pump!

Once you've adopted the Pump way of life, you are set for life. We truly believe you will have a happier, healthier life if you eat and live within the tenets of the Pump. Keep up your exercise routine, which shouldn't be a hardship because, since you already work out regularly, you feel more energized, sleep better, feel less stressed, and have fewer aches and pains. Avoid all those nasty wrong foods and become increasingly creative and adventuresome with the right ones. Take a look at our recipes for ideas.

Never hesitate to get advice or help from doctors, nutritionists, and trainers. The doctor will make sure you are healthy enough to start a program of diet and exercise. The nutritionist will help you plan a sensible regimen of vitamins and supplements. If you aren't taking vitamins now, it's generally advisable to take less than suggested on the label until your body has developed a tolerance. Talk about this with your nutritionist. Finally, the right trainer can help you use your time at the gym more efficiently for optimal benefits and little risk of injury.

Now that you have made the commitment, are eating healthfully and well, and are enjoying all the wonderful recipes on the following pages, you are part of the Pump solution. There still will be times when you are confused about food choices. Let us help.

To stay true to the Pump, don't eat protein, carbohydrates, and cheese at the same time.

HERE ARE SOME SPECIFIC EXAMPLES OF COMBINATIONS TO AVOID:

- cheeseburgers (skip the cheese and the bun)
- pizza with pepperoni (order a vegetarian thin-crust pizza with very little cheese)
- cheese steak with fries (try a simple grilled steak)
- lasagna (cheese, pasta, and meat is the worst combination you can eat)
- egg and cheese sandwiches on a bagel (try an egg white omelet)
- spinach pie (remove and discard the extra dough)

We also recommend forgoing some common menu items, regardless of how much you like them.

THESE ARE GOOD EXAMPLES OF BAD CARBOHYDRATES:

- pancakes with syrup
- cinnamon rolls
- doughnuts
- muffins

As you eat your three daily meals, plus snacks (Chapter 14) and shakes (Chapter 10), remember to eat twice as much of a vegetable as a protein—and make sure the protein is a good protein. Dress salads with a low-fat dressing (we have some terrific ones in Chapter 11).

Remember, reaching your goal and committing to eating and living healthfully is the best feeling in the world. A great body doesn't come in a pill or a bottle, and you can't buy one.

It's up to you. Take it from us, it's not as hard to get there as you may think, and once you do, the sky is the limit!

How to Use This Book

As you use this cookbook, whether recipe by recipe or by employing one of the two-week diet and eating plans included toward the back, pay attention to the codes next to each recipe. We have indicated whether each recipe is particularly helpful for staying energized, losing weight, building muscle, or getting into shape. Many of the recipes can help you do all four. The icons next to each recipe have the following meanings:

HAVE ENERGY

STAY FIT

LOSE WEIGHT

BUILD MUSCLE

The icons are meant to guide you as you work to achieve your weight loss and/or fitness goals, but if you have a particular craving, you should feel free to eat outside the codes within this book. We created all of these recipes with healthful eating in mind, and the absence of a particular icon next to a recipe does not mean that the recipe will have an adverse effect on your goals.

The Pump provides by far the finest quality, best-tasting food we have found anywhere outside of our own cooking. This food is perfectly engineered. Lean protein, complex carbohydrates, and essential fats—your body needs all of these, plain and simple. Your eating habits should be a lifestyle. That is what the Pump is all about; it is a way of life. We have done hundreds of interviews for magazines and television and the most asked question is "What do you think of all these diets out there?" Our answer is plain and simple: "Not much." Diet is a short-term solution to a bigger problem. Your eating habits should be a Lifestyle. That is what the Pump is all about; it is a way of life. Take care of your body from the inside out. The esthetics will follow and you will be much healthier for it.

—KENNEDY & STROM FITNESS, INC.

www.ksfitness.com

02.
Appetizers

Guacamole the Pump Way / Chunky Oil-Free Avocado Salsa / Pumped-Up Hummus / The Pump's
Baked Falafel / Baked Cauliflower Appetizer / Herbed Shallot-Stuffed Portobello Mushrooms / Cheese-Topped
Baked Portobello Mushrooms

Guacamole the Pump Way

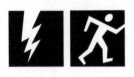

WE MAKE OUR GUACAMOLE WITHOUT ADDED OIL, SO IT'S NEVER HEAVY, and while avocados contain fat, it's a healthful fat. These rich, lush fruits can be expensive, so it's a good idea to mix them with cucumbers and scallions to stretch them. That way you also get the flavor without too many calories. Increase the cayenne pepper and add a fresh jalapeño if you like spicier guacamole. Buy avocados a few days before you use them and let them ripen on the countertop (never in the refrigerator!). Handle with care, as they bruise easily. We love dipping grilled chicken or steak in our guacamole or mixing it with cooked beans.

MAKES ABOUT 3 CUPS

4 **AVOCADOS**, peeled and pitted

1 large or 2 small **CUCUMBERS**, peeled, seeded, and roughly chopped (about 1⅓ cups)

JUICE OF 2 SMALL LIMES

½ cup chopped **SCALLIONS**, white and green parts

½ cup firmly packed chopped fresh **CILANTRO**

1 teaspoon extra-virgin **OLIVE OIL**

1 small **GARLIC** clove, minced

⅛ teaspoon **CAYENNE PEPPER**

Pinch of **SEA SALT**, optional

In the bowl of a food processor fitted with the metal blade, combine the avocados, cucumbers, lime juice, scallions, and cilantro. Pulse just until mixed and chunky.

Add the olive oil, garlic, and cayenne. Season to taste with salt, if using. Process until nearly smooth but with a little texture. Serve immediately or transfer to a small glass bowl and cover with plastic wrap resting directly on the surface of the guacamole. Refrigerate for up to 1 day. Leaving an avocado pit in the guacamole will help keep it fresh.

NUTRITIONAL ANALYSIS (per 2-tablespoon serving):
Total carbohydrates: 2 g / Protein: 0 g / Fat: 2 g / Dietary fiber: 1 g / Calories: 25

Chunky Oil-Free Avocado Salsa

SURE, AVOCADOS ARE PRETTY HIGH IN FAT, BUT IT'S A GOOD FAT and a little goes a long way in the satisfaction department. Plus, they taste wonderful. Make sure the avocado is ripe before you make this salsa. Leave hard, unripe fruit on the kitchen counter for a day or more for it to ripen. It's ready when it gives when you press it gently. Eat this as a snack, spooned over chicken or fish, or on a sandwich. No oil, no guilt!

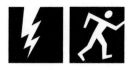

MAKES ABOUT 4 1/2 CUPS

2 ripe **AVOCADOS**, pitted, peeled, and cut into
  1/2- to 1-inch chunks
1 seedless **CUCUMBER**, peeled and cut into
  1/2-inch cubes (about 2 cups)
2 medium **TOMATOES**, peeled and coarsely
  chopped

1 small **JALAPEÑO**, seeded and minced
1 small clove **GARLIC**, crushed, optional
3 tablespoons minced fresh **CILANTRO**
3 to 4 tablespoons fresh **LIME JUICE**

A realistic, comprehensive, appetizing menu for the health-conscious person.
—MARK G. COHEN, Cardiologist
MD, FACC, FACP

In a small glass bowl, combine the avocados, cucumber, tomatoes, jalapeño, garlic, if using, and cilantro. Mash and toss with a fork to mix well. Add 3 tablespoons of lime juice, taste, and add more if needed. Leave the salsa chunky, not smooth.

NUTRITIONAL ANALYSIS (per 2-tablespoon serving):
Total carbohydrates: 1 g / Protein: 0 g / Fat: 1.5 g / Dietary fiber: 1 g / Calories: 15

Pumped-Up Hummus

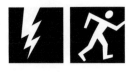

SOME BODYBUILDERS USE HUMMUS LIKE OTHER PEOPLE USE BUTTER. They spread it on everything! And why not? Chickpeas are full of fiber, protein, and complex carbohydrates, which help boost your natural immunity. Like most things, hummus is much better if you make it yourself; you know exactly what goes into it, and with a food processor, it's easy, easy, easy. Make a batch of this, add more or less paprika and cumin to suit your taste, and keep it in the refrigerator for up to three days, which we think is as long as most foods should be stored.

MAKES ABOUT 2 3/4 CUPS

2 1/2 cups cooked or canned and drained **CHICKPEAS**, see page 107

2 1/2 tablespoons **TAHINI**

1/2 teaspoon **SWEET PAPRIKA**

1/2 teaspoon ground **CUMIN**

1/2 teaspoon **GARLIC POWDER**

1/4 teaspoon freshly ground **BLACK PEPPER**

1/2 bunch **FLAT-LEAF PARSLEY**, coarsely chopped (about 1 cup)

JUICE OF 1 LEMON

1/2 cup diced **ONION**

Pinch of **SEA SALT**, optional

4 to 5 tablespoons **WATER**

In the bowl of a food processor fitted with the metal blade, combine the chickpeas, tahini, paprika, cumin, garlic powder, pepper, parsley, and lemon juice. Process for about 30 seconds until blended. Add the onion and a tiny pinch of salt, if using. Pulse until mixed and nearly smooth.

Taste the hummus and add as much water as necessary for the correct consistency. Process until as smooth as you like.

Serve the hummus at once or transfer to a glass or plastic container with a tight-fitting lid and refrigerate for up to 3 days. Let the hummus reach room temperature before serving.

NOTE: If using canned, well-rinsed chickpeas, omit the salt completely.

NUTRITIONAL ANALYSIS (per 2-tablespoon serving):
Total carbohydrates: 5 g / Protein: 2 g / Fat: 1.5 g / Dietary fiber: 1 g / Calories: 35

The Pump's Baked Falafel

BAKING THIS FLAVORFUL CHICKPEA MIXTURE RATHER THAN FRYING IT results in a healthful treat without the grease. Delicious with hummus or tahini—great for a party.
SERVES 16

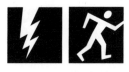

½ pound dried **CHICKPEAS**
OLIVE OIL COOKING SPRAY
2 tablespoons **TAHINI**
1 **ROMAINE LETTUCE HEART**,
    roughly chopped
2 medium **ONIONS**, coarsely chopped
¼ cup fresh **LEMON JUICE**

1 tablespoon **OLIVE OIL**, optional
1 clove **GARLIC**, minced
1 teaspoon **CUMIN**
½ teaspoon **GROUND CORIANDER**
½ teaspoon **WHITE PEPPER**
½ teaspoon **SEA SALT**, optional

Rinse the chickpeas under cool water. Transfer to a bowl and add enough cold water to cover by 1 or 2 inches. Refrigerate for 24 hours. Drain, and let the chickpeas dry completely in a colander. They must be dry to make the falafel. You should have about 3 cups of chickpeas.

Preheat the oven to 425°F. Lightly spray a baking sheet with olive oil cooking spray.

In the bowl of a food processor fitted with the metal blade, process the chickpeas and tahini until finely chopped but not completely smooth. Remove from the food processor and set aside.

Without rinsing the bowl, put the lettuce and onion in the food processor and pulse 7 to 8 times or until finely chopped. Scrape from the bowl and add to the chickpeas.

Add the lemon juice, olive oil, if using, garlic, cumin, coriander, and pepper. Stir, mixing the chickpeas well with the other ingredients. Add the salt, if using.

Form the falafel into small balls by packing the mixture firmly into 1-ounce scoops or a similar small container. Arrange the balls on the baking sheet. You will have between 48 and 64 balls. Bake for about 15 minutes or until lightly browned and heated through. The balls will be soft. Serve warm.

NUTRITIONAL ANALYSIS (per serving):
Total carbohydrates: 20 g / Protein: 6 g / Fat: 2.5 g / Dietary fiber: 4 g / Calories: 120

Baked Cauliflower Appetizer

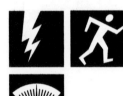

HAVING FRIENDS OVER? Make this and serve it with Guacamole the Pump Way (page 14) or our Pumped-Up Hummus (page 16).p You'll never miss the chips. They are absolutely wonderful, and as they bake they develop a nice crispness. A big winner!

SERVES 6

1 head **CAULIFLOWER**, broken into florets, tough stems discarded (about 1 pound of florets)

1 tablespoon **DRIED PARSLEY-ONION MIX**, such as Mrs. Dash
1 teaspoon **LEMON PEPPER**
OLIVE OIL COOKING SPRAY

Preheat the oven to 375°F.

Put the florets in a large bowl and sprinkle with the parsley-onion mix and lemon pepper. Spray lightly with olive oil spray and toss to mix.

Spread the cauliflower florets in a single layer in a shallow baking pan.

Bake for 25 minutes, turning once. Reduce the oven temperature to 300°F and bake for 15 to 20 minutes longer, turning once, until lightly golden and a little crispy. Serve warm.

NUTRITIONAL ANALYSIS (per serving):
Total carbohydrates: 4 g / Protein: 1 g / Fat: .5 g / Dietary fiber: 2 g / Calories: 20

Herbed Shallot-Stuffed Portobello Mushrooms

WE STAY AWAY FROM BREAD, BUT we have a weakness for classic tomato-basil bruschetta, such as is served in Italian restaurants. Using large, flat portobello mushrooms is a good way to avoid the bread but still get the fantastic flavors of sun-ripened tomatoes, summer's best basil, fruity olive oil, and a splash of white balsamic vinegar. You will make this over and over again. We do!

SERVES 6

OLIVE OIL COOKING SPRAY

6 medium **PORTOBELLO MUSHROOMS**, stemmed (5 to 6 ounces each)

1 large **SHALLOT**, finely chopped

1 large **TOMATO**, cored and chopped

15 to 20 large **FRESH BASIL LEAVES**, chopped

1 teaspoon extra-virgin **OLIVE OIL**

1 teaspoon **WHITE BALSAMIC VINEGAR**

SEA SALT, optional

Preheat the oven to 425°F. Spray a baking sheet or baking pan with olive oil cooking spray.

Wipe the mushrooms with a clean, dry towel. Lay the mushrooms on the tray and spray with a little more cooking spray.

Bake for 20 to 30 minutes, turning the mushrooms once during baking, or until the mushrooms are soft and tender.

Meanwhile, in a small mixing bowl, stir together the shallot, tomato, and basil leaves. Stir in the olive oil, vinegar, and a tiny pinch of sea salt, if using. You will have about 1½ cups of topping.

When the mushrooms are soft, remove them from the oven. Spoon a little of the topping onto the mushroom caps, spreading it over the inside of the caps. Serve immediately.

NUTRITIONAL ANALYSIS (per serving):

Total carbohydrates: 6 g / Protein: 2 g / Fat: 2.5 g / Dietary fiber: 2 g / Calories: 60

As a photographer, I recommend The Pump all the time to the male and female models and actors I shoot. For lean, "pumped" physiques they need high protein, low fat fuel. No added salt means less puffiness in the face and no added sugar translates to fewer mood swings. The vast menu offers so many truly great tasting choices, from protein rich energy charged plates to a variety of healthful indulgences. And, it seems they're always coming up with new creative innovations. I find the Pump is a much shared secret within the fitness, modeling, and acting worlds.

—PETER D. BROWN

Cheese-Topped Baked Portobello Mushrooms

FOR A TRULY WONDERFUL INDULGENCE, try this the next time you have company. It's great when you crave cheese. We are partial to mushrooms, and big, glorious portobellos can stand up to baking. Buy large, flat mushrooms.

SERVES 4

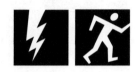

OLIVE OIL COOKING SPRAY
4 **PORTOBELLO MUSHROOMS**, stemmed
4 **PLUM TOMATOES**, cored and thinly sliced
1 teaspoon dried **BASIL**

Freshly ground **BLACK PEPPER** to taste
½ cup shredded low-fat **MOZZARELLA** or
   SOY CHEESE

Preheat the oven to 375°F. Spray a shallow baking pan with olive oil cooking spray.

Arrange the mushrooms, gill sides up, in the pan and bake for about 15 minutes. Turn the mushrooms over and cook for 15 to 20 minutes longer or until soft. Remove from the oven and turn the mushrooms over so that gill sides face up again.

Lay the tomato slices on top of the mushrooms. Bake for 10 to 12 minutes or until the tomatoes soften.

Sprinkle the mushrooms and tomatoes with basil and pepper and top with shredded cheese. Bake for 3 to 5 minutes longer or until the cheese melts. Serve right away.

NUTRITIONAL ANALYSIS (WITH LOW-FAT MOZZARELLA, PER SERVING):
Total carbohydrates: 10 g / Protein: 19 g / Fat: 7 g / Dietary fiber: 2 g / Calories: 180

03.
Soups and Sandwiches

The Pump Chicken Soup / Tofu–Vegetable Soup / Butternut Squash Soup / Carrot–Sweet Potato Soup / Lentil Soup / Dynamite Pita Sandwich / Grilled Lemon Chicken Sandwich / Chicken and Spinach Sandwich / The New York Sandwich / Tuna Salad Sandwich with Hummus / Vegetarian Special Sandwich

The Pump Chicken Soup

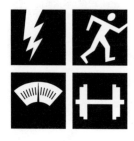

IT'S THE NUMBER OF VEGETABLES THAT MAKES THIS SOUP OUR FAVORITE and incredibly popular with our customers. It doesn't have the fat and starch of other chicken soups (no rice, no pasta), and the flavor is sublime. The herbs are crucial to the final result, but use the amount we suggest. Too many herbs will muddy the flavor. We use lemon peel in place of salt for a bright, fresh flavor. For an even lighter soup, cook the chicken separately and add the meat to the soup just before serving. For richer chicken flavor, cook it as described here. We like it with white meat only, but you can make it with both white and dark meat. For a vegetarian soup, substitute tofu for the chicken. If you work out, you could eat nothing but this soup for a couple of days, lose weight, and develop muscle tone. How great is that?

SERVES 14

2 tablespoons **OLIVE OIL**, optional

1 pound **YELLOW ONIONS**, chopped

4 ribs **CELERY**, sliced on the diagonal

1 pound **CARROTS** (about 5 medium carrots), trimmed, peeled, and sliced on the diagonal

1/2 pound **PARSNIPS** (2 medium parsnips), peeled, halved if large, and sliced on the diagonal

8 stems **FLAT-LEAF PARSLEY**

4 stems fresh **THYME**

4 large leaves **FRESH SAGE**

2 stems fresh **MARJORAM**

1 strip **LEMON PEEL**, colored part only, about 4 inches long and 1/2 inch wide

3 1/2 quarts **WATER**

3 pounds **CHICKEN BREASTS** or one 3-pound **CHICKEN**, split or cut into 8 pieces, or 1 package of chicken parts

1 teaspoon **SEA SALT**, optional

1/2 teaspoon freshly ground **BLACK PEPPER**, optional

NOTE: Olive oil can help preserve the soup for up to three days. If you will be eating the soup on the first or second day, then it is unnecessary.

In a stockpot, heat the olive oil, if using, over low heat. Add the onions and celery and cook, stirring, for about 5 minutes or until softened. Add the carrots and parsnips and cook, stirring occasionally to prevent sticking, for 4 to 5 minutes longer or until the vegetables begin to soften.

Using kitchen twine, tie the parsley, thyme, sage, marjoram, and lemon peel in a bundle. You could also wrap the herbs and lemon peel in a piece of cheesecloth, fold it into a package, and tie it closed with kitchen twine.

Add the water, chicken, herb bundle, and salt and pepper, if using, to the pot; raise the heat and bring to a boil over high heat. Reduce the heat and simmer gently, partially covered, for about 35 minutes or until the chicken is cooked through. The internal temperature of white meat should be 160°F and of dark meat, 180°F.

Lift the chicken from the pot and set aside to cool for about 20 minutes. Let the vegetables continue to simmer gently in the broth.

When the chicken is cool enough to handle, remove and discard the bones and skin. Chop the meat into bite-size pieces. You will have about 2 cups of chopped chicken.

Remove and discard the herb bundle. Add the chicken to the stockpot and stir and cook gently for 3 to 5 minutes or until heated through. Serve hot.

NUTRITIONAL ANALYSIS (per serving):
Total carbohydrates: 11 g / Protein: 24 g / Fat: 2.5 g / Dietary fiber: 2 g / Calories: 160

Tofu-Vegetable Soup

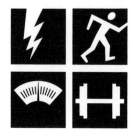

WE THINK OF THIS SOUP AS A BIG BOWL OF HEALTH! The tofu and vegetables are nutritious, and while the list of ingredients for this soup is long, you can eat a generous serving and never feel bloated or overfed. You will actually be bursting with energy. Tofu, a soy product, is a great source of protein. If you can't find one of the vegetables listed below, buy a similar one—for example, rutabaga for turnips or yellow onions for sweet onions.

SERVES 8

8 cups **WATER**

4 ribs **CELERY**, chopped

3 large **VIDALIA** or other **SWEET ONIONS**, chopped and rinsed with cool water

2 **PARSNIPS**, peeled and sliced (about ¾ cup)

1 **LEEK**, trimmed and chopped

1 small **PURPLE-TOPPED TURNIP** (about 4 ounces), coarsely diced

1 clove **GARLIC**, minced

½ pound **CARROTS**, peeled and chopped

1 large bunch fresh **DILL**, chopped (about 1 cup)

1 bunch **FLAT-LEAF PARSLEY**, chopped (about 1 cup)

¼ cup **DRY WHITE WINE**, optional

14 to 16 ounces **FIRM** or **EXTRA-FIRM TOFU**, drained and cut into ½-inch cubes (about 3 cups)

Freshly ground **BLACK PEPPER**

SEA SALT, optional

In a large saucepan, bring the water to a boil over high heat.

Add the celery, onions, parsnips, leek, turnip, garlic, carrots, dill, parsley, and wine, if using, and return to a boil. Reduce the heat and simmer the soup for 20 to 30 minutes, stirring occasionally, or until the vegetables are tender.

Add the tofu and heat over low heat for about 5 minutes, or until heated through.

Taste the soup and adjust the seasoning with pepper. If you want to add salt, do so just before serving for the best flavor.

NUTRITIONAL ANALYSIS (per serving):

Total carbohydrates: 15 g / Protein: 8 g / Fat: 4 g / Dietary fiber: 4 g / Calories: 120

Butternut Squash Soup

HERE'S A GOOD EXAMPLE OF HOW THE RIGHT COMBINATION OF VEGETABLES can make a satisfying, thick soup with little effort. While some cooks might add cream, butter, or reduced beef stock to enrich this soup, we stir it as it cooks so it has time to develop body and flavor. If you like butternut squash, you will love this soup.

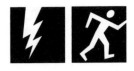

SERVES 6

1 medium **BUTTERNUT SQUASH** (about 2 pounds)

3 **VIDALIA** or other **SWEET ONIONS**, finely chopped and rinsed with cool water

6 ounces **BABY CARROTS**, peeled and chopped (about 1 1/4 cups)

4 ribs **CELERY**, halved lengthwise and chopped

2 **TURNIPS**, peeled, halved, and chopped

1/2 cup chopped fresh **DILL** (1/2 bunch), plus 2 tablespoons for garnish

6 cups **WATER**

3 tablespoons **OLIVE OIL**

1/2 teaspoon **SEA SALT,** optional

NONFAT PLAIN YOGURT for garnish, optional

Cut the squash into large pieces, peel, and scoop out the seeds. Chop the cleaned squash into small, bite-size pieces.

In a large pot with a cover, cook the onions over medium heat for about 5 minutes to soften and until the onions release their juices. Add the carrots, cover the pot, and cook for about 5 minutes longer until the carrots begin to soften. Add the chopped squash, celery, turnips, dill, and water. Stir in the olive oil and season to taste with salt, if needed.

Bring to a boil over medium-high heat, reduce the heat slightly, and simmer, partially covered, for about 40 minutes, stirring frequently, or until the vegetables are soft and the flavors blend. Serve hot and garnish each bowl with a dollop of yogurt if desired and a sprinkling of chopped dill.

NOTE: This soup is best made a few hours or a day ahead of time, refrigerated, and then reheated.

NUTRITIONAL ANALYSIS (without plain nonfat yogurt, per serving):
Total carbohydrates: 30 g / Protein: 3 g / Fat: 7 g / Dietary fiber: 7 g / Calories: 180

Carrot-Sweet Potato Soup

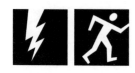

THE FIRST TIME STEVE MET ELENA'S PARENTS, HER MOTHER, a confirmed vegetarian, made carrot soup. It was different from this one but made a lasting impression. Ours is made with sweet potatoes as well, for a lovely, rich-tasting soup that proves you don't need oil or salt for a smooth, soothing soup. Sweet potatoes provide an extra burst of energy—an added bonus. We once tried to take it off the menu at the Pump—just to give it a rest—but our customers rose up in protest!

SERVES 8

1 pound **ONIONS**, roughly chopped (about 3½ cups)

6 cups **WATER**

1½ pounds **SWEET POTATOES**, peeled and roughly chopped (2 to 3 potatoes; about 4½ cups)

½ pound **CARROTS**, peeled and roughly chopped (about 1½ cups)

2 teaspoons finely grated **ORANGE ZEST**

NONFAT PLAIN YOGURT for garnish, optional

Fresh **DILL**, chopped, for garnish

Put the onions and ½ cup of the water in a heavy stockpot, cover tightly, and cook over low heat for 12 to 15 minutes, stirring occasionally until softened.

Add the sweet potatoes, carrots, orange zest, and the remaining water and bring to a simmer. Cook, partially covered, over medium-low heat for 45 to 50 minutes, or until the potatoes and carrots soften.

Transfer the soup to a blender or food processor and puree. You will have to do this in batches. Alternatively, use an immersion blender to puree the soup directly in the pan.

Serve the soup garnished with a dollop of yogurt, if desired, and garnished with dill.

NUTRITIONAL ANALYSIS (per serving):
Total carbohydrates: 25 g / Protein: 3 g / Fat: 0 g / Dietary fiber: 5 g / Calories: 110

Lentil Soup

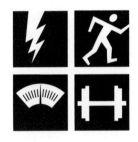

THE FIRST TIME STEVE SAW ANYONE USE SOUP AS A DRESSING was about twenty-five years ago, when he watched a trainer spoon lentil soup over a pita bread sandwich. What a great idea! Of course, this is equally delicious as soup. You'll never go wrong eating lentil soup—the lentils are good for you and full of iron, and the soup is warm and nourishing in every way.

SERVES 12

10 cups **WATER**
2 pounds **ONIONS**, peeled and chopped (about 5 cups)
6 ribs **CELERY**, chopped (about 2¼ cups)
2¼ pounds **PLUM TOMATOES**, diced (about 3 cups)
1 pound **CARROTS**, peeled and shredded (about 3 cups)

1 pound dried **LENTILS**
½ teaspoon **SEA SALT**, optional
¼ teaspoon freshly ground **BLACK PEPPER**, optional
½ cup minced **FLAT-LEAF PARSLEY**
2 tablespoons **OLIVE OIL**, optional

In a large, heavy stockpot, put ¼ cup of water. Add the onions and celery, cover, and cook over low heat, stirring or shaking the pan occasionally, for about 15 minutes or until softened. Add the tomatoes and carrots and cook over medium-low heat for 15 to 20 minutes.

Add the remaining water and the lentils, bring to a simmer over medium heat, add the olive oil, if using, and cook, partially covered, for 50 to 60 minutes or until the lentils are tender.

Season with salt and pepper, if using, stir in the parsley, and serve hot.

NOTE: Olive oil can help preserve the soup for up to three days. If you will be eating the soup on the second or third day, be sure to add it.

NUTRITIONAL ANALYSIS (per serving):
Total carbohydrates: 31 g / Protein: 12 g / Fat: .5 g / Dietary fiber: 14 g / Calories: 170

Dynamite Pita Sandwich

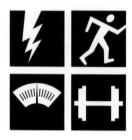

THIS SANDWICH MAY BE ONE OF THE MOST DELICIOUS and healthful sandwiches ever made. It includes nothing you shouldn't eat, and yet it's a true taste treat. No cheese, no fat, just chicken and tomatoes and a little burst of hummus.

SERVES 1

2 tablespoons seeded and minced **TOMATO**

1 tablespoon minced **ONION**

1 tablespoon minced **GREEN BELL PEPPER**

2 tablespoons **THE PUMP'S HOMEMADE TOMATO SAUCE**, page 110

5 to 6 ounces cooked boneless, skinless **CHICKEN BREAST**, lean **SIRLOIN STEAK**, or **NATURE BURGER**, page 117, see Note

1 tablespoon **PUMPED-UP HUMMUS**, page 16

1 whole wheat 7-inch **PITA BREAD**, lightly toasted

In a small bowl, toss together the tomato, onion, and pepper. Add the tomato sauce and stir to mix. Transfer the vegetables to a nonstick skillet and warm over medium-high heat for 8 to 10 minutes or until heated through.

Let the cooked meat come to room temperature, if it has been refrigerated. Add to the vegetables and mix well.

Spoon the hummus over the pita and spoon the tomato-meat mixture over the hummus. Fold the pita and serve.

NOTE: If you start with uncooked meat, broil or grill it in a countertop grill, such as a George Foreman Grill, for 6 to 8 minutes for the chicken or until cooked through, and 5 to 6 minutes for the steak for medium rare.

NUTRITIONAL ANALYSIS (per serving):
Total carbohydrates: 41 g / Protein: 41 g / Fat: 6 g / Dietary fiber: 6 g / Calories: 370

Grilled Lemon Chicken Sandwich

WITH THE SALAD, CHICKEN, AND PITA, THIS SANDWICH IS PERFECTLY BALANCED
with enough fiber and protein for an easy and light meal. Spice up this recipe with a lively oil and vinegar dressing with herbs. It tastes great with any of our dressings; choose your favorite.

SERVES 1

3 to 4 tablespoons **PUMP SALAD**, without dressing, page 38

1 whole wheat 7-inch **PITA BREAD**, halved to make 2 pockets

1 cooked **CHICKEN BREAST** from Grilled Lemon Chicken, page 91, cut into 6 slices

1 tablespoon **OIL AND VINEGAR DRESSING WITH HERBS**, page 171

Spoon the salad into the pita bread pockets. Add the chicken and spoon the dressing over the chicken. Serve immediately.

NUTRITIONAL ANALYSIS (per serving):
Total carbohydrates: 38 g / Protein: 39 g / Fat: 7 g / Dietary fiber: 5 g / Calories: 350

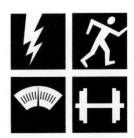

I love the Pump! I started eating there three years ago, and I'm so glad I did. I was living on Staten Island, and I used to love going to the city to get a Dynamite Pita Sandwich. When I finally moved to Manhattan, I made sure to [find an] apartment near the Pump. I love how it makes me feel. I can eat a lot and still feel healthy. I am a singer and my appearance is important. The Pump helps me stay looking great while allowing me to chow down on great-tasting meals.

—TYRA, singer

Chicken and Spinach Sandwich

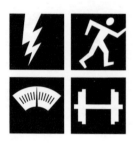

OUR CUSTOMERS LOVE THIS ONE! And with one bite you'll understand why it's one of our most popular sandwiches. All the ingredients work well together, and there's nothing to object to in terms of healthful eating—or in terms of flavor!

SERVES 1

3 ounces **SPINACH LEAVES**, rinsed (about 3 cups)

1 small cooked boneless, skinless **CHICKEN BREAST** (about 5 to 6 ounces) or **ROASTED WHITE MEAT TURKEY**, cut into 5 to 6 slices

1 whole wheat 7-inch **PITA BREAD**

1 tablespoon **PUMP HOMEMADE TOMATO SAUCE**, page 110, or your favorite tomato sauce

3 ounces nonfat **MOZZARELLA**, shredded

Preheat the oven to 425°F.

In a steamer basket set over boiling water or in an electric steamer, steam the spinach for about 1 minute or until wilted. Lift the spinach from the basket and set aside to cool slightly. Drain if necessary.

Put the chicken or turkey in the pita bread and top with the spinach. Spoon the tomato sauce over the spinach and top with the cheese. Press the pita closed and put in a small baking pan. Toast for 3 to 4 minutes or until the cheese melts and the sandwich is heated through. Serve hot.

NUTRITIONAL ANALYSIS (per serving):
Total carbohydrates: 39 g / Protein: 67 g / Fat: 5 g / Dietary fiber: 9 g / Calories: 450

The New York Sandwich

WE CALL THIS THE NEW YORK BECAUSE, LIKE OUR CITY, the sandwich is big and bold, full of gusto and flavor. Make it with chicken, steak, or a Nature Burger, whichever fits your diet and meets your fancy.

SERVES 1

5 to 6 ounces cooked boneless, skinless
  CHICKEN BREAST or lean **SIRLOIN STEAK**,
  sliced, or a **NATURE BURGER**, page 117,
  see Note
3 tablespoons **PUMPED-UP HUMMUS**, page 16
1 whole wheat 7-inch **PITA BREAD**,
  toasted and split open

ROMAINE LETTUCE LEAVES, torn into pieces
1 tablespoon chopped **TOMATO**
2 teaspoons minced **RED ONION**
3 to 4 slices **CUCUMBER**

Let the meat come to room temperature if it's been refrigerated.

Spread the hummus inside the pita bread. Lay the chicken, steak, or burger on top of the hummus and stuff the pita with lettuce, tomato, onion, and cucumber slices. Fold over the sandwich and serve immediately.

NOTE: If you start with uncooked meat, broil or grill it in a countertop grill for 6 to 8 minutes for the chicken or until cooked through, and 5 to 6 minutes for the steak for medium rare.

NUTRITIONAL ANALYSIS (per serving):
Total carbohydrates: 36 g / Protein: 41 g / Fat: 7 g / Dietary fiber: 6 g / Calories: 350

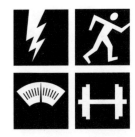

The guys here at the gym love the Pump. Their delivery people must come here five times a day. I especially like the #42, turkey burger on a pita with tomatoes, onions, and hummus. The tomatoes are amazingly fresh and I love their tahini sauce.
—RICK B., Definitions

Good nutrition is just as important as a good workout. That's why I go to the Pump. Try #61, Iron.
—ALAN, Definitions

Tuna Salad Sandwich with Hummus

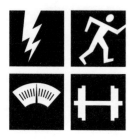

IF YOU LIKE TUNA SANDWICHES IN GENERAL, YOU WILL LOVE THIS ONE! We avoid fat-laden mayonnaise, instead tossing the tuna with hummus. Eat this for lunch for a great protein boost and indescribable flavor.

SERVES 1

1 6-ounce can **WHITE ALBACORE TUNA**, packed in water

2 tablespoons **PUMPED-UP HUMMUS**, page 16

1 **WHOLE WHEAT 5-INCH PITA BREAD**, toasted and split

3 to 4 tablespoons **PUMP SALAD** with dressing, page 38

1½ tablespoons **OIL AND VINEGAR DRESSING WITH HERBS**, page 171, optional

Drain the tuna and transfer to a small bowl. Flake the tuna with a fork. Add the Pumped-Up Hummus and stir until well mixed.

Carefully spoon the tuna-hummus mixture into the pita bread. Stuff the sandwich with Pump Salad. Add more salad, if desired. Drizzle with the dressing, if desired, and serve immediately.

NUTRITIONAL ANALYSIS (per serving):
Total carbohydrates: 29 g / Protein: 26 g / Fat: 4.5 g / Dietary fiber: 4 g / Calories: 260

Vegetarian Special Sandwich

THIS SANDWICH IS SERVED WARM WITH MELTED CHEESE, and as such is satisfying as only a toasted sandwich can be. It can be a substantial snack or a light meal. Serve it with a cup of lentil soup for a full, balanced meal.

SERVES 1

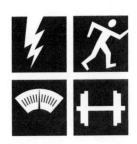

1 cup sliced **BROCCOLI** florets

1 cup peeled and sliced **CARROTS** (3 to 4 ounces)

1 whole wheat 7-inch **PITA BREAD**

3 ounces nonfat **MOZZARELLA** or **SOY CHEESE**, shredded (about 1 cup)

1 tablespoon **CARROT-GINGER DRESSING**, optional, page 174

Preheat the oven to 425°F.

In a steamer basket set over simmering water or in an electric steamer, steam the broccoli and carrots for 1 to 2 minutes, or until tender. Remove the vegetables from the steamer and set aside to cool slightly. Drain if necessary.

Spoon the vegetables into the pita bread and top with the cheese. Press the pita closed and put in a small baking pan. Toast for 3 to 4 minutes or until the cheese melts and the sandwich is heated through. Top with the dressing, if desired, and serve hot.

NOTE: Substitute steamed cauliflower, zucchini, or spinach for the broccoli and carrots.

NUTRITIONAL ANALYSIS (per serving):
Total carbohydrates: 43 g / Protein: 35 g / Fat: 1.5 g / Dietary fiber: 11 g / Calories: 320

04.
Salads

Pump Salad / Tomato–Basil Salad with Thyme Vinaigrette / Tuna Salad with Soy Mayonnaise / Classic Green Salad / Romaine Dill Salad / Our Favorite Salad / Three-Bean Salad / Five-Vegetable Salad / Cucumber Salad / Cucumber and Watercress Salad / Green Cabbage Salad / Red Cabbage Salad with Black-Eyed Peas / Greek Salad / Beautiful and Delicious Chickpea Salad / Green Leaf Lettuce Salad with Cilantro / Salad Finale with Cilantro and Red Beans / Asparagus Salad / Fresh Artichoke Salad / String Bean Salad / Red Kidney Bean Salad with Fresh Tomatoes / Black Bean and Corn Salad / French Bean and Tomato Salad

Pump Salad

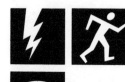

IF A RESTAURANT DOESN'T HAVE A GOOD SALAD, WALK OUT. We think it's a good indication of the freshness of the rest of the food. This salad is our flagship salad, and you can't find a more refreshing and straightforward one anywhere. Plus, it's easy to make, with ingredients always available in the markets. Tomatoes are best in the summertime, but in the colder months, look for small plum tomatoes, cherry tomatoes, or on-the-vine tomatoes (which can be a little pricey). We spoon this salad, dressed or not, into pita bread sandwiches and also offer it as a chopped salad. If you prefer, make it as a leafy side salad (see the variation at the end of the recipe). Either way, it's green, fresh, and crispy.

SERVES 4

1 **ROMAINE LETTUCE HEART**, chopped into small pieces

1 medium **CUCUMBER**, peeled and chopped

½ medium **RED ONION**, chopped

1 medium **TOMATO**, cored, seeded, and chopped

3 to 4 tablespoons **OIL AND VINEGAR DRESSING WITH HERBS**, page 171

In a mixing bowl, toss the chopped lettuce, cucumber, onion, and tomato. Drizzle with dressing and toss to mix. Serve immediately.

VARIATION: For a more traditional, leafy salad, tear the lettuce into pieces, slice the cucumber into rounds, cut the onion into strips, and slice the tomato into thin rounds. Toss the vegetables, except the tomato, and then toss with the dressing. Arrange the tomato slices on top of the salad or decoratively around the rim of the bowl or platter.

NUTRITIONAL ANALYSIS (per serving):
Total carbohydrates: 8 g / Protein: 1 g / Fat: 1.5 g / Dietary fiber: 2 g / Calories: 45

Tomato-Basil Salad with Thyme Vinaigrette

FOR US, THE MARRIAGE OF TOMATOES AND BASIL MAKES LIFE BETTER—no matter what else is going on. This salad is especially good in the summertime, when tomatoes are at their best and rinsing red onions under cool, running water cuts their sharpness. We prefer frisée, which is tart and crunchy, but use another green if you like.

SERVES 6

4 ripe unblemished **SUMMER TOMATOES** (about 1 pound)

1 small **RED ONION**, sliced

3 tablespoons extra-virgin **OLIVE OIL**

2 tablespoons freshly squeezed **LEMON JUICE**

1 tablespoon **BALSAMIC VINEGAR**

2 teaspoons minced fresh **THYME LEAVES**

2 small bunches **FRISÉE (CURLY ENDIVE)**, rinsed and spun dry

12 large **BASIL LEAVES**, torn into pieces

18 **KALAMATA** or **GAETA PITTED OLIVES**, rinsed and halved

Pinch of **SEA SALT**, optional

Core the tomatoes and slice them into thin wedges. Transfer to a glass bowl.

Rinse the onion slices under cool, running water to remove their sharpness. Set aside to dry on paper towels. Add to the bowl with the tomatoes.

Meanwhile, in a small bowl, whisk together the oil, lemon juice, vinegar, and thyme. (This vinaigrette keeps for up to 2 days if covered and refrigerated.)

Add the frisée, basil leaves, and olives to the bowl with the tomatoes. Toss and dress with the vinaigrette. Season with salt, if desired. Serve immediately.

NUTRITIONAL ANALYSIS (per serving):
Total carbohydrates: 14 g / Protein: 3 g / Fat: 11 g / Dietary fiber: 6 g / Calories: 160

Tuna Salad with Soy Mayonnaise

WE LIKE TUNA PACKED IN WATER; IF YOU PREFER TUNA in oil, buy it packed in water and then add your own olive oil. It will taste better and you can control the amount. Soy mayonnaise is sold in health food stores, and once you try it, you'll love it. Trust us! It's an easy, filling dish full of protein and fresh vegetables—as good for a light meal as for a snack.

SERVES 4

Two 6-ounce cans water-packed **SOLID WHITE ALBACORE TUNA**
3 ribs **CELERY**, finely chopped
1 medium **ONION**, finely chopped

3 tablespoons **SOY MAYONNAISE**
Sliced **TOMATOES**
CELERY STICKS

In a small bowl, flake the tuna with a fork.

Add the celery, onion, and mayonnaise and stir to mix. Serve with sliced tomatoes and celery sticks.

NUTRITIONAL ANALYSIS (per serving):

Total carbohydrates: 7 g / Protein: 22 g / Fat: 6 g / Dietary fiber: 1 g / Calories: 170

About one year ago I had the good fortune of having a Pump Energy Food eatery move in just around the corner from my office. As a chiropractor, I am constantly teaching my patients about health and wellness, and to have this golden example of healthy, tasty food at my fingertips was a blessing. Not only did the Pump provide me with a well-balanced food option, it gave me the chance to show my patients how food should be prepared, eaten, and enjoyed.
—CHRIS ANSELMI, chiropractor

One of my clients has gained 50 pounds of solid muscle by eating at the Pump three times per day and he's a vegetarian. Another client has lost 40 pounds of fat by eating low glycemic foods that don't leave him bingeing at night and he's more energetic and positive than ever.

I tell my clients not to be afraid of food, especially those wanting to shed fatty pounds. Good food is your ticket to burning body fat and maintaining quality muscle. You can have a great body and eat great food too.

—GENNARO FERRA, personal fitness trainer / former Mr. Australia
www.gennaroferra.com

Classic Green Salad

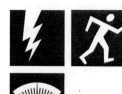

EATING GREENS WITH PROTEIN IS ONE OF THE KEYS TO DIETARY SUCCESS because greens help your body break down proteins. We believe in eating the right foods together. For instance, if you crave a burger, go ahead, but serve it on a bed of greens or with tomatoes. Forget the French fries and bun!

SERVES 4

1 large head **RED LEAF LETTUCE**, washed, spun dry, and torn into pieces

16 to 20 **CHERRY TOMATOES**, stem marks removed, halved

1/4 large **VIDALIA** or other **SWEET ONION**, chopped and rinsed in cool water

4 tablespoons extra-virgin **OLIVE OIL**

2 tablespoons **BALSAMIC VINEGAR**

SEA SALT and freshly ground **PEPPER**, optional

In a large mixing bowl, toss the lettuce with the tomatoes and onion. Drizzle the olive oil and vinegar over the vegetables and toss to mix. Season to taste with salt and pepper, if desired. Serve immediately on salad plates.

NUTRITIONAL ANALYSIS (per serving):
Total carbohydrates: 7 g / Protein: 2 g / Fat: 14 g / Dietary fiber: 2 g / Calories: 160

Romaine Dill Salad

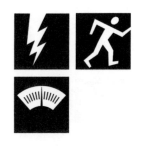

ROMAINE LETTUCE IS NEARLY ALWAYS AVAILABLE and its crispness improves any salad—especially this simple one. Dill, with its grassy flavor, is also great in this salad. It stimulates the taste buds, and due to its distinctive flavor, you don't need salt with the salad. The white balsamic vinegar provides lovely, clean flavor.

SERVES 6

1 large or 2 small **ROMAINE LETTUCE HEARTS**, coarsely chopped
1 small bunch fresh **DILL**, chopped
½ cup thinly sliced **SCALLIONS**

2 tablespoons white **BALSAMIC VINEGAR**
1 tablespoon extra-virgin **OLIVE OIL**
Chopped fresh **OREGANO**

In a large bowl, toss the lettuce with the dill and scallions.

In a small bowl, whisk together the vinegar and oil. Pour over the greens and toss to mix. Sprinkle a little oregano over the salad and serve immediately.

NUTRITIONAL ANALYSIS (per serving):
Total carbohydrates: 5 g / Protein: 2 g / Fat: 2.5 g / Dietary fiber: 2 g / Calories: 50

Our Favorite Salad

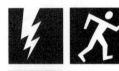

WE'VE GIVEN THIS SALAD OUR HIGHEST PRAISE, calling it our favorite because it's chunky, filling, and refreshing. The soft, tender tomatoes and avocados are perfect with crispy cucumbers and onions for an overall outstanding salad experience!

SERVES 12

SALAD:
5 medium **TOMATOES**, cored, peeled, and sliced
5 **AVOCADOS**, peeled, pitted, and sliced
4 large **CUCUMBERS**, peeled, halved lengthwise, and sliced into half moons, about 1/4 inch thick
1 small **RED ONION**, cut into thin wedges and rinsed in cool water

DRESSING:
1/3 cup extra-virgin **OLIVE OIL**
1/3 cup **WHITE WINE VINEGAR**
2 teaspoons dried **CELERY FLAKES**, crushed
1 tablespoon chopped fresh or dried **LEMONGRASS** or grated **LEMON ZEST**, see Note

Arrange the tomatoes on a large platter and top with the avocados. Top with the cucumbers and onion.

In a small bowl, whisk together the olive oil and vinegar. Crush the celery flakes between your fingers and discard any hard pieces. Add to the dressing with the lemongrass. Whisk just until mixed. Pour over the vegetables and serve immediately.

NOTE: Fresh lemongrass is widely available in all markets. Dried lemongrass is found in the spice section at some supermarkets. A jar contains three or four 3-inch pieces, which must be reconstituted in warm water before using.

NUTRITIONAL ANALYSIS (per serving):
Total carbohydrates: 15 g / Protein: 3 g / Fat: 19 g / Dietary fiber: 7 g / Calories: 220

Three-Bean Salad

WHEN A DISH LOOKS AS PRETTY AS THIS ONE DOES, it just tastes better! We nearly always have this salad in our refrigerator. It's great with chicken, fish, or beef, and we like to spoon it over brown rice, too. It will perk up any meal.

SERVES 10

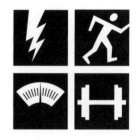

2¼ to 2½ cups cooked **BLACK BEANS** (1 cup before cooking), see Note

2¼ to 2½ cups cooked **WHITE BEANS** (1 cup before cooking), see Note

2¼ to 2½ cups cooked **RED KIDNEY BEANS** (1 cup before cooking), see Note

½ cup diced **RED ONION**

⅓ cup diced **YELLOW BELL PEPPER**

½ bunch **CILANTRO**, chopped (about ⅔ cup loosely packed)

½ cup **WHITE WINE** or **SHERRY VINEGAR**

⅓ cup extra-virgin **OLIVE OIL**

¼ cup fresh **LEMON JUICE**

½ teaspoon **SEA SALT**, optional

In a large mixing bowl, combine the beans, onion, pepper, and cilantro. Toss to mix.

In a small bowl, whisk together the vinegar, olive oil, and lemon juice. Season to taste with salt, if desired. Pour the dressing over the beans, toss well, and set aside at room temperature for about 30 minutes for the flavors to blend. This salad can be refrigerated for up to 1 day but tastes best on the day it is made. Bring to room temperature before serving for the best flavor.

NOTE: For directions on how to cook dried beans, see the box on page 107.

NUTRITIONAL ANALYSIS (per serving):
Total carbohydrates: 30 g / Protein: 11 g / Fat: 8 g / Dietary fiber: 9 g / Calories: 240

Five-Vegetable Salad

A FRESH SIDE SALAD DOES NOT NEED LETTUCE TO BE CRISPY AND REFRESHING. Try this salad with the summer's best tomatoes; sweet carrots; crispy, crunchy cucumbers and peppers; and sweet, tangy red onion slices. The mustardy dressing brings the flavors together.

SERVES 6

3 large **TOMATOES**, stemmed and chopped (about 1½ pounds)

1 large seedless **CUCUMBER**, peeled and sliced into rounds

1 **CARROT**, shredded

⅔ cup diced **ORANGE BELL PEPPER**

½ cup thinly sliced **RED ONION**

MUSTARD-THYME VINAIGRETTE, page 173

In a mixing bowl, toss together the tomatoes, cucumber, carrot, bell pepper, and onion. Drizzle the dressing over the salad and toss to coat. Serve immediately.

NUTRITIONAL ANALYSIS (per serving):
Total carbohydrates: 4 g / Protein: 1 g / Fat: 7 g / Dietary fiber: 1 g / Calories: 80

Cucumber Salad

WE RECOMMEND EATING THIS SIMPLE CUCUMBER SALAD WITH FISH. Its lightness and fresh-ness complement nearly any white-fleshed fish, such as halibut and flounder, and it's a natural fit with oilier fish, such as salmon.

SERVES 6

3 large **CUCUMBERS**, peeled and sliced (about 5 cups)

½ medium **RED ONION**, diced

¾ teaspoon dried **OREGANO**

¾ teaspoon dried **BASIL**

2 tablespoons extra-virgin **OLIVE OIL**

2 tablespoons **WHITE BALSAMIC VINEGAR**

Pinch of **SEA SALT**, optional

In a mixing bowl, toss the cucumbers, onion, oregano, and basil.

In a small bowl, whisk together the oil and vinegar. Pour over the cucumbers and onion, toss gently, season to taste with salt, if desired, and serve within 30 minutes of preparing.

NUTRITIONAL ANALYSIS (per serving):
Total carbohydrates: 7 g / Protein: 1 g / Fat: 5 g / Dietary fiber: 1 g / Calories: 70

Cucumber and Watercress Salad

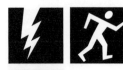

THIS IS A TERRIFIC SALAD BECAUSE IT'S MADE WITH PEPPERY WATERCRESS, a lively green that makes any salad better. Watercress is easy to find in the springtime, but you can usually locate it all year long. We combine the watercress with cucumbers, red onions (made milder by rinsing in cool water), orange peppers, and white mushrooms.

SERVES 6

6 ounces **WATERCRESS**, rinsed, thick stems removed and discarded

2 **CUCUMBERS**, peeled, halved lengthwise, and sliced into half moons

1/2 **RED ONION**, thinly sliced and rinsed with cool water

1/2 **ORANGE BELL PEPPER**, diced

10 ounces **WHITE MUSHROOMS**, chopped

1/4 cup **WHITE BALSAMIC VINEGAR**

3 tablespoons **OLIVE OIL**

JUICE OF 1 LIME

3 tablespoons minced **FRESH TARRAGON LEAVES**

1/4 teaspoon **SEA SALT**, optional

Mince the watercress leaves and transfer to a bowl. Add the cucumbers, onion, pepper, and mushrooms.

In a small mixing bowl, whisk together the vinegar and oil. Add the lime juice, tarragon, and salt, if using. Whisk again and then drizzle over the salad. Toss well to mix. Serve immediately.

NUTRITIONAL ANALYSIS (per serving):
Total carbohydrates: 9 g / Protein: 2 g / Fat: 7 g / Dietary fiber: 1 g / Calories: 110

Green Cabbage Salad

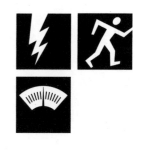

THIS SALAD IS INCREDIBLE. Green cabbage makes a salad with good volume. It's inexpensive, and as a cruciferous vegetable, is known to protect against certain types of cancer. For a filling, complete meal, toss this salad with a can of tuna.

SERVES 6

1 small head **GREEN CABBAGE** (about 2½ pounds), outer leaves removed and discarded

3 tablespoons **OLIVE OIL**

2 tablespoons **RICE WINE VINEGAR**

SEA SALT, optional

Halve the cabbage head and remove the core. Thinly slice, as you would for coleslaw. Transfer the cabbage to a mixing bowl.

Add the olive oil and vinegar and toss to coat. Season to taste with salt, if desired.

NUTRITIONAL ANALYSIS (per serving):
Total carbohydrates: 11 g / Protein: 2 g / Fat: 7 g / Dietary fiber: 4 g / Calories: 120

Red Cabbage Salad with Black-Eyed Peas

RED CABBAGE IS COLORFUL, AND WHEN MIXED WITH BLACK-EYED PEAS, it forms an interesting and healthful salad. Add a can of tuna and this salad turns into a substantial main course, but even without the tuna, it's filling and nutritious. Sprinkle a handful of nutty brown rice over the salad to add crunch. Just this small amount of rice provides the satisfaction that, on a different eating plan, croutons might.

SERVES 8

2 cups cooked **BLACK-EYED** or **YELLOW PEAS**, see box on page 106

2 **CUCUMBERS**, peeled, seeded, and chopped

2 **CARROTS**, shredded

1/2 small head **RED CABBAGE**, chopped

1/2 **GREEN BELL PEPPER**, chopped

4 **SCALLIONS**, white and green parts, thinly sliced

5 tablespoons **WHITE BALSAMIC VINEGAR**

4 tablespoons extra-virgin **OLIVE OIL**

1 tablespoon **MUSTARD SEEDS**

1 tablespoon **SWEET PAPRIKA**

1/2 teaspoon **SEA SALT,** optional

1/4 cup minced **FLAT-LEAF PARSLEY**, optional

In a mixing bowl, toss together the peas, cucumbers, carrots, cabbage, pepper, and scallions. In a small mixing bowl, whisk together the vinegar and olive oil.

Lightly crush the mustard seeds in a mortar with a pestle and add to the oil and vinegar. Add the paprika and salt, if using, whisk well, and drizzle over the salad. Toss well and serve immediately. Garnish with parsley.

NUTRITIONAL ANALYSIS (per serving):
Total carbohydrates: 19 g / Protein: 3 g / Fat: 8 g / Dietary fiber: 5 g / Calories: 150

Greek Salad

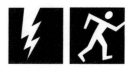

OUR FAVORITE PART OF ANY GREEK SALAD IS THE FETA CHEESE. Not everyone likes it, but if you buy good sheep or goat feta, preferably from a Greek market or top-grade cheese counter, you might surprise yourself. We rinse the feta before slicing it to wash away some of the salt and then store it in fresh, cold water in the refrigerator. We compare feta to avocados: A little of either goes a long way, but both are so good! A pinch of oregano perks up the flavor of this salad, which is a natural complement to lamb. For a full meal, serve this with grilled chicken or legumes such as white beans.

SERVES 6

1 large head **ROMAINE LETTUCE**

1/2 large or 1 small **VIDALIA** or other **SWEET ONION**, julienned or sliced thin (about 1 cup), rinsed with cool water

2 medium **CUCUMBERS**, peeled and cut into wedges

8 ounces **FETA CHEESE**, cubed

1 teaspoon dried **OREGANO**

1/4 cup **OLIVE OIL**

2 tablespoons **WHITE WINE VINEGAR**, optional

1/2 teaspoon **SEA SALT**, optional

Remove and discard the outer leaves of the head of romaine lettuce. Chop the lettuce and transfer to a colander. There should be about 8 cups. Rinse under cold water, shake or spin dry, and set aside to drain completely.

In a salad bowl, combine the rinsed onion, cucumber, and feta. Add the lettuce and oregano. Toss with the olive oil and vinegar, if using. Season to taste with salt, if desired. Serve immediately.

NUTRITIONAL ANALYSIS (per serving):
Total carbohydrates: 9 g / Protein: 9 g / Fat: 5 g / Dietary fiber: 2 g / Calories: 240

Beautiful and Delicious Chickpea Salad

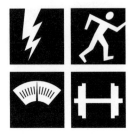

DEPENDING ON HOW MUCH YOU EAT, THIS SALAD CAN BE AN APPETIZER, main course, or side salad. Chickpeas are great sources of fiber and protein, but beyond their healthfulness, they taste good and have great texture. You never feel you're eating healthy when you make this salad.
SERVES 6

2½ cups cooked or canned and drained
   CHICKPEAS, see box on page 107
1 **RED** or **GREEN BELGIUM ENDIVE**, chopped
1 **CARROT**, shredded
¼ medium **GREEN BELL PEPPER**, finely
   chopped

½ bunch **FLAT-LEAF PARSLEY**, chopped
½ cup **WHITE BALSAMIC VINEGAR**
¼ cup **OLIVE OIL**
SEA SALT, optional

In a nonreactive bowl, toss the chickpeas, endive, carrot, pepper, and parsley.

In a small mixing bowl, whisk together the vinegar and olive oil. Season to taste with salt, if desired.

Immediately toss the vegetables with the dressing to prevent the endive from discoloring. Serve immediately or cover and refrigerate for up to 2 days.

NUTRITIONAL ANALYSIS (per serving):
Total carbohydrates: 23 g / Protein: 6 g / Fat: 11 g / Dietary fiber: 6 g / Calories: 220

Green Leaf Lettuce Salad with Cilantro

THIS GREEN SALAD IS SIMILAR TO OTHERS WE LIKE, but the cilantro gives it a sunny flavor and makes it especially good with chili and other foods with Mexican flavors. The cucumbers provide body and crunch, and if you can't find green leaf lettuce, use red leaf instead.

SERVES 6

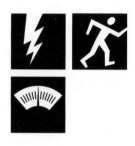

1 head **GREEN** or **RED LEAF LETTUCE**

2 **TOMATOES**, cored and quartered

1 large **CUCUMBER**, peeled, sliced horizontally, and sliced into half moons

1/2 **RED ONION**, sliced into thin strips

1/2 **ORANGE BELL PEPPER**, sliced into thin strips

2/3 cup chopped fresh **CILANTRO**

1/4 cup extra-virgin **OLIVE OIL**

2 tablespoons fresh **LEMON JUICE**

Pinch of dried **OREGANO**

SALT and freshly ground **BLACK PEPPER**, optional

Tear the head of lettuce into leaves, rinse well, dry, and tear the leaves into large pieces.

In a mixing bowl, toss together the lettuce, tomatoes, cucumber, onion, pepper, and cilantro.

In a small mixing bowl, whisk together the olive oil, lemon juice, oregano, and salt and pepper, if using, to taste. Drizzle over the salad. Toss well and serve immediately.

NUTRITIONAL ANALYSIS (per serving):
Total carbohydrates: 7 g / Protein: 2 g / Fat: 10 g / Dietary fiber: 1 g / Calories: 120

Salad Finale with Cilantro and Red Beans

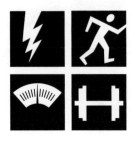

RED BEANS HAVE FIRMER TEXTURE AND A LITTLE MORE DISTINCT FLAVOR than chickpeas, which is one reason we like them here. This salad can be a first course, main dish, or side dish, but whichever way you serve it, it's highly nutritious with protein (from the beans) for energy and only complex carbohydrates. How can you go wrong?

SERVES 8

2 cups cooked or canned and drained
    RED KIDNEY BEANS, see box on page 107
1/2 head **GREEN CABBAGE**, coarsely shredded
    (about 5 cups)
1/2 **RED ONION**, sliced
1/2 **ORANGE BELL PEPPER**, diced
1 bunch fresh **CILANTRO**, large stems
    discarded, leaves chopped (about 1 cup)

JUICE OF 2 LIMES
6 tablespoons **WHITE BALSAMIC VINEGAR**
3 tablespoons extra-virgin **OLIVE OIL**
1/4 teaspoon **SEA SALT**, optional
2 large **TOMATOES**, cored and cut into
    thin slices
2 **AVOCADOS**, peeled, pitted, and diced

In a mixing bowl, toss together the beans, cabbage, onion, pepper, and cilantro. Set aside 2 tablespoons of lime juice.

In a small mixing bowl, whisk together the vinegar, olive oil, remaining lime juice, and salt, if using. Drizzle over the salad and toss well.

Arrange the tomato slices on a serving platter. Spoon the bean and cabbage salad over the tomatoes.

Toss the avocados with the reserved 2 tablespoons of lime juice. Spoon over the salad and serve immediately.

NUTRITIONAL ANALYSIS (per serving):
Total carbohydrates: 22 g / Protein: 6 g / Fat: 13 g / Dietary fiber: 9 g / Calories: 220

Asparagus Salad

WHEN STEVE WAS YOUNG, HE NEVER LIKED ASPARAGUS, BUT ONE DAY he had lunch with a bodybuilder friend who ordered it and then raved about its nutritional properties and great taste. Since then, we've learned that asparagus is a valuable source of beta-carotene and vitamins B and C. These days, we both love it and eat it all year long, but especially in the spring, when all the markets carry it and it's fresh and not too expensive.

SERVES 8

2 bunches **ASPARAGUS SPEARS** (about 2 pounds)

4 **TOMATOES**, cored and cut into wedges

2 **CUCUMBERS**, peeled and chopped into 1½-inch chunks

1 bunch **SCALLIONS**, white and green parts, sliced

1 bunch **WATERCRESS**, rinsed, thick stems removed and discarded

¼ cup **WHITE BALSAMIC VINEGAR**

2 tablespoons extra-virgin **OLIVE OIL**

½ teaspoon **PAPRIKA**

½ teaspoon freshly ground **BLACK PEPPER**

Fresh **LIME JUICE**, optional

SEA SALT, optional

Cut the tips from the asparagus into 2-inch lengths. Reserve the stalks for another use. In an electric steamer or steamer basket set over an inch or so of boiling water, steam the asparagus tips for 1 to 2 minutes or until tender. Set aside to cool.

Transfer the asparagus tips to a serving bowl. Add the tomatoes, cucumbers, scallions, and watercress and toss to mix.

In a small bowl, whisk together the vinegar, olive oil, paprika, and pepper. Drizzle over the salad and toss well. Season to taste with lime juice or salt, if desired.

NUTRITIONAL ANALYSIS (per serving):
Total carbohydrates: 12 g / Protein: 4 g / Fat: 4 g / Dietary fiber: 1 g / Calories: 90

Fresh Artichoke Salad

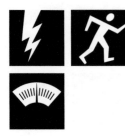

IF YOU'RE IN THE MOOD FOR SOMETHING SPECIAL, ARTICHOKES WILL FIT THE BILL. Steve recalls eating them when he was a child growing up in Greece, where they were steamed, cooled, and tossed with a vinegar-based dressing. Here we toss them with a lemony dressing and serve them with olives and parsley for a salad that hearkens back to Steve's Greek roots. It's wonderful as a lunch dish.

SERVES 6

SALAD:
2 large fresh **ARTICHOKES**
1 slice of **LEMON**
2 to 3 tablespoons fresh **LEMON JUICE**
4 **CUCUMBERS**, peeled and sliced
About 25 **GRAPE TOMATOES** (about 5 ounces), halved
1/2 **GREEN BELL PEPPER**, seeded and diced

DRESSING:
1/2 cup fresh **LEMON JUICE**
GRATED ZEST OF 1 LEMON
2 tablespoons extra-virgin **OLIVE OIL**
Pinch of **SALT**, optional
Freshly ground **BLACK PEPPER**
8 green **COLOSSAL OLIVES**, pitted and slivered (about 1/4 cup)
1 medium **CARROT**, peeled and shredded
1/4 cup minced **FLAT-LEAF PARSLEY**

Cut a thin slice from the stem end of the artichokes to freshen them. Put in a large pot that holds them snugly. Add the lemon slice and enough cold water to come 2 inches up the side. Cover tightly and bring the water to a boil over medium-high heat. Reduce the heat to low and simmer gently for 25 to 30 minutes, or until the base of the artichokes are tender when pierced with the tip of a sharp knife.

Plunge the artichokes in a bowl filled with ice water to halt cooking. Drain upside down in a colander for 20 to 30 minutes or until cool enough to handle.

Remove the outer leaves from both artichokes. Cut off the stems and continue to remove the leaves until you uncover the inedible, fuzzy chokes. Cut it away to expose the hearts of the artichokes. Rub each artichoke heart with lemon juice.

In a large bowl, toss the cucumber slices, grape tomatoes, and bell pepper.

Slice the artichoke hearts and add to the bowl.

In a small bowl, whisk together the lemon juice, lemon zest, and olive oil. Season with a tiny pinch of salt, if using, and pepper to taste. Pour the dressing over the salad and toss gently to mix.

Sprinkle the olives, shredded carrot, and parsley over the salad and serve.

NUTRITIONAL ANALYSIS (per serving):

Total carbohydrates: 14 g / Protein: 3 g / Fat: 6 g / Dietary fiber: 5 g / Calories: 110

String Bean Salad

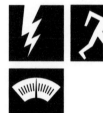

WE LOVE STRING BEANS, COOKED JUST UNTIL CRISPY TENDER. They have an earthy flavor and a marvelous bite. Here we toss them with a lovely, light, fresh-tasting dressing made from white balsamic vinegar and lemon juice and just a tablespoon of extra-virgin olive oil. Let this salad sit for about 30 minutes for the flavors to develop and serve it at room temperature. You'll love it! **SERVES 4**

1 pound **STRING BEANS**, washed, trimmed, and left whole or halved if very long
½ **RED ONION**, thinly sliced
½ cup diced **ORANGE BELL PEPPER**
3 tablespoons **WHITE BALSAMIC VINEGAR**
2 tablespoons fresh **LEMON JUICE**

1 tablespoon extra-virgin **OLIVE OIL**
1 teaspoon dried **BASIL**
Pinch of **SEA SALT**, optional

In an electric steamer or a steamer basket set over boiling water, steam the beans for 3 to 5 minutes, or until al dente. Cool slightly and transfer to a mixing bowl.

Rinse the onion slices under cool, running water to remove their sharpness. Set aside to dry on paper towels. Add to the bowl with the string beans and the pepper.

Sprinkle the vinegar, lemon juice, olive oil, and basil over the vegetables. Toss to mix and season with salt, if desired. Let the salad rest for about 30 minutes to allow the flavors to blend. Serve at room temperature.

NUTRITIONAL ANALYSIS (per serving):
Total carbohydrates: 13 g / Protein: 2 g / Fat: 3.5 g / Dietary fiber: 4 g / Calories: 90

Red Kidney Bean Salad with Fresh Tomatoes

WE THINK RED BEANS LOOK SO PRETTY WITH TOMATOES that we serve this often during the summer, when vine-ripened tomatoes are delicious and juicy. The beans are a good source of protein, so while this salad is a wonderful side, you can also serve it as a main course. Keep it refrigerated and eat it within two or three days.

SERVES 5

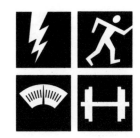

1/2 small **RED ONION**, thinly sliced

5 tablespoons **WHITE BALSAMIC VINEGAR**

3 tablespoons extra-virgin **OLIVE OIL**

1/4 teaspoon **SEA SALT**, optional

2 cups cooked **RED BEANS**, see box on page 107

2 **TOMATOES**, cored and sliced into thin wedges

3/4 cup seeded and thinly sliced **YELLOW BELL PEPPER**

1/2 cup minced **FLAT-LEAF PARSLEY**

Rinse the sliced onion under cool, running water, drain, and pat dry with paper towels.

In a small bowl, whisk together the vinegar, olive oil, and salt, if using.

In a mixing bowl, combine the beans, onion, tomatoes, and bell pepper. Add the dressing and toss to mix. Add the parsley, toss, and serve.

NUTRITIONAL ANALYSIS (per serving):

Total carbohydrates: 24 g / Protein: 7 g / Fat: 9 g / Dietary fiber: 6 g / Calories: 200

Black Bean and Corn Salad

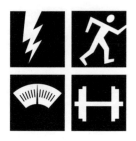

DURING THE SUMMER, WHEN THE CORN IS SWEET AND PLENTIFUL, we make this salad all the time. The recipe produces a lot of salad, which is intentional, since it keeps for a few days and can be combined with meat, chicken, or grilled fish for an even more substantial meal.

SERVES 14

8 ears fresh **CORN**

6 1/2 cups cooked or drained and rinsed
   BLACK BEANS, see box on page 107

3 tablespoons diced **RED ONION**

1/2 cup **WHITE BALSAMIC VINEGAR**

1/4 cup extra-virgin **OLIVE OIL**

Juice of 1 **LIME**

1 teaspoon ground **CUMIN**

1/2 teaspoon **CAYENNE PEPPER**, or more to taste

3 large **PLUM TOMATOES**, seeded and
   chopped (about 3/4 pound)

1 **AVOCADO**, peeled and cut into 3/4-inch
   chunks

1/2 cup packed chopped fresh **CILANTRO**

Preheat the oven to 375°F.

Pull the husks from the ears without detaching them. Remove the silk and pull the leaves back over the corn and fold closed. Lay the ears of corn in a single layer on 1 or 2 baking pans. Bake for about 25 minutes, turning the ears once, until the husks turn light brown. The kernels will turn a deeper shade of golden yellow.

Let the corn cool in their husks. Remove the husks and slice the kernels from the corncobs. To do so, stand the cobs on end on a plate or cutting board and using a small, sharp knife slice the kernels off the cob.

In a large mixing bowl, stir together the corn, black beans, and onion.

In another small bowl, whisk together the vinegar, olive oil, lime juice, cumin, and cayenne. Pour the dressing over the salad and toss to mix.

Just before serving, add the tomatoes, avocado, and cilantro and toss gently.

NUTRITIONAL ANALYSIS (per serving):

Total carbohydrates: 42 g / Protein: 10 g / Fat: 7 g / Dietary fiber: 9 g / Calories: 250

French Bean and Tomato Salad

FRENCH BEANS, ALSO CALLED HARICOTS VERTS, ARE LONG AND SLENDER. Any pole bean works here, which is why we also suggest yellow wax beans or ordinary green beans. This salad is colorful, elegant enough to serve at a dinner party as a side dish without the rice. With the rice, it's a refreshing main course.

SERVES 4

2 large **PLUM TOMATOES**, cored, seeded, and diced

1/2 cup diced **YELLOW BELL PEPPER**

1/3 cup diced **VIDALIA** or other **SWEET ONION**

2 teaspoons minced fresh **OREGANO** or **TARRAGON**

2 tablespoons **OLIVE OIL**

2 tablespoons **SHERRY VINEGAR** or **TARRAGON VINEGAR**

SEA SALT, optional

1/2 pound slender **GREEN BEANS**, **WAX BEANS**, or **HARICOTS VERTS**, trimmed

2 cups cooked **BROWN RICE**, see box on page 139

In a small mixing bowl, combine the tomatoes, pepper, and onion and sprinkle with oregano or tarragon. Drizzle the olive oil and vinegar over the vegetables and toss to mix. Season to taste with salt, if desired. Set aside while you steam the beans.

In a steamer basket set over boiling water or in an electric steamer, steam the beans for 3 to 4 minutes or until tender (steam 1 to 2 minutes if cooking haricots verts).

Drain, and using tongs, arrange on a serving platter. Top with the tomato mixture and serve with brown rice.

NUTRITIONAL ANALYSIS (per serving):
Total carbohydrates: 35 g / Protein: 4 g / Fat: 8 g / Dietary fiber: 4 g / Calories: 230

05.
Fish and Seafood

Broiled Scallops with Paprika / Pan-Seared Scallops with Tomatoes and Parsnips / Lemon-Dill Shrimp / Shrimp with Capers / Halibut with Fresh Ginger / Baked Salmon with Tomato Salsa / Baked Salmon with Cauliflower and Lemon Sauce / Fillet of Flounder with Pesto

Broiled Scallops with Paprika

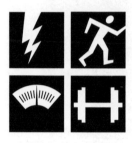

SCALLOPS ARE ELEGANT AND LIGHT AND ARE NEVER BETTER than when broiled perfectly so that they are soft and tender on the inside and lightly crunchy on the outside. We season them with lemon and paprika for an elegant meal that goes best with a glass of wine and candlelight. Buy creamy-looking sea scallops from a merchant you trust. They must be fresh with virtually no odor. Avoid scallops that are bright, bright white, which means they have been soaked in a preservative solution. While harmless, the solution dilutes the scallop's already delicate flavor.

SERVES 4

OLIVE OIL COOKING SPRAY
$1^{1}/_{2}$ pounds **SEA SCALLOPS**
Juice of 2 **LEMONS**

$1/_2$ cup of **WATER**
1 tablespoon **SWEET PAPRIKA**

Preheat the broiler. Spray a broiling pan with olive oil cooking spray.

Rinse the scallops under cold water and pat dry with paper towels. Lay the scallops in a single layer on the broiling pan and broil 2 inches from the heat source for 4 to 5 minutes, turning at least once, until lightly browned and cooked through and opaque. The scallops will cook quickly and should be watched closely.

Meanwhile, mix together the lemon juice, water, and paprika. Drizzle lemon juice sauce over each serving of hot scallops. Pass any leftover sauce on the side.

NUTRITIONAL ANALYSIS (per serving):
Total carbohydrates: 2 g / Protein: 40 g / Fat: 3 g / Dietary fiber: 0 g / Calories: 200

Pan-Seared Scallops with Tomatoes and Parsnips

YOU NEVER FEEL YOU'RE MISSING OUT ON GOOD FOOD when scallops are on the menu!
SERVES 6

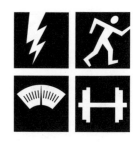

JUICE OF 1 LEMON

1½ tablespoons finely grated **LEMON ZEST**

2 tablespoons fresh **THYME LEAVES**

¼ teaspoon **SEA SALT,** optional

2 pounds **SEA SCALLOPS**

2 tablespoons **OLIVE OIL**

2 large **ONIONS**, chopped

½ **YELLOW BELL PEPPER**, seeded and diced

6 large **PLUM TOMATOES**, chopped (about 3 cups)

2 small **PARSNIPS**, peeled and diced (about 3 cups)

1 cup **WATER**

OLIVE OIL COOKING SPRAY

¼ cup minced **FLAT-LEAF PARSLEY**

In a small bowl, stir together the lemon juice and zest, thyme, and salt, if using. Remove 2 tablespoons of the lemon mixture.

Toss the scallops with the 2 tablespoons of the lemon mixture. Set aside to marinate slightly while the stew cooks.

Meanwhile, in a large saucepan, heat the oil over medium-high heat. Add the onions and pepper and cook for 3 to 4 minutes until they begin to soften. Add the tomatoes, parsnips, and water, bring to a simmer, reduce the heat to low, cover, and cook for 30 minutes, stirring every 4 or 5 minutes, until the parsnips are tender and the mixture is nicely blended.

Place 2 large skillets (preferably cast iron) over medium-high heat and spray lightly with cooking spray.

Drain the scallops and pat them dry with paper towels. Divide the scallops between the hot skillets and cook for about 2 minutes just until the scallops begin to brown. Turn the scallops and cook for 1 to 2 minutes longer or until golden brown, cooked through, and opaque.

Divide the stewed vegetables evenly among 6 bowls. Top with the seared scallops. Garnish with parsley.

NUTRITIONAL ANALYSIS (per serving):
Total carbohydrates: 19 g / Protein: 37 g / Fat: 7 g / Dietary fiber: 4 g / Calories: 290

Lemon-Dill Shrimp

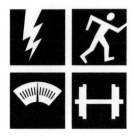

DILL AND SHRIMP ARE A NATURAL PAIRING, and when you add lemon juice, the flavors dance. Who can resist their sweet flavor for too many weeks at a time? We recommend buying them in the shell, which makes them less expensive; they also tend to be fresher. If you submerge the unpeeled shrimp in water, they are easier to peel.

SERVES 4

2 pounds unpeeled **LARGE SHRIMP**

JUICE OF 3 LEMONS

4 tablespoons **DRIED PARSLEY-ONION MIX**,
    such as Mrs. Dash

12 to 15 sprigs of fresh **DILL**, coarsely chopped

Preheat the broiler.

Put the shrimp in a bowl and cover with water. This makes peeling easier. Peel and devein the shrimp. Rinse with cold water, drain, and put in a single layer in a broiling pan.

Pour the lemon juice over the shrimp and sprinkle with the parsley-onion mix. Broil 5 to 6 inches from the heat for 6 to 8 minutes, turning several times, until the shrimp are pink and cooked through.

Remove the shrimp from the broiler. Scatter the dill over the shrimp. Cover pan with aluminum foil for about 3 minutes to keep the shrimp warm and give the flavors time to blend. Serve immediately with any pan juices spooned over the shrimp.

NUTRITIONAL ANALYSIS (per serving):
Total carbohydrates: 3 g / Protein: 36 g / Fat: 2 g / Dietary fiber: 0 g / Calories: 180

Shrimp with Capers

WHEN YOU MIX SWEET SHRIMP WITH SALTY CAPERS, you create a tasty dish but not one that is so salty that you feel thirsty an hour after eating. We use lime juice here, which works well with the capers, but you could substitute lemon juice, too. The sun-dried tomatoes provide another texture and round out the flavor of these broiled gems. Serve this with the Asparagus Salad on page 55 for an outstanding meal!

SERVES 4

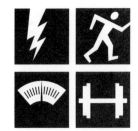

2 pounds unpeeled **LARGE SHRIMP**
1/2 cup **DRY WHITE WINE**
2 tablespoons **OLIVE OIL**
JUICE OF 2 LARGE OR 3 SMALL LIMES

1/3 cup drained **CAPERS**
SEA SALT, optional
14 **SUN-DRIED TOMATOES**, halved or
    quartered if large

I am 33 years old. My 60-year-old father and I are planning to run the New York Marathon together. We [plan] to eat Pump foods to prepare us. I have loved the Pump for years and know that it gives such great energy. We will need it!
—TRICIA KELLY

Preheat the broiler.

Put the shrimp in a bowl and cover with water. This makes peeling easier. Peel and devein the shrimp and transfer to another bowl.

Add the wine, olive oil, all but 1 tablespoon of the lime juice, and capers. Mix gently and set aside to marinate for about 10 minutes.

Spread the shrimp in a broiling pan. Pour the accumulated juices and capers over the shrimp.

Broil the shrimp 5 to 6 inches from the heat and cook for 4 minutes. Turn the shrimp and broil for about 3 to 4 minutes longer, or until the shrimp are pink and cooked through. Season with remaining tablespoon of lime juice, if desired, and a sprinkling of salt. Garnish with sun-dried tomatoes.

NUTRITIONAL ANALYSIS (per serving):
Total carbohydrates: 5 g / Protein: 37 g / Fat: 10 g / Dietary fiber: 1 g / Calories: 280

Halibut with Fresh Ginger

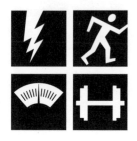

FIRM, MILD, AND LEAN, HALIBUT IS ONE OF THE BEST WHITE OCEAN FISH you can eat. We cook this with a little fresh ginger for a taste you will want to revisit again and again. This recipe is a good example of how fish should be cooked: simply and without a lot of flourishes.

SERVES 4

OLIVE OIL COOKING SPRAY

1½ pounds **HALIBUT FILLET**, cut into
   4 pieces

JUICE OF 1 LARGE LEMON (about 2/3 cup)

2 tablespoons **OLIVE OIL**

1 tablespoon freshly grated **GINGER**

1 tablespoon chopped fresh **THYME LEAVES**

Freshly ground **BLACK PEPPER** and
   SEA SALT, optional

Preheat the oven to 425°F.

Spray a baking pan large enough to hold the halibut in a single layer with cooking spray. Lay the halibut in the pan.

In a small bowl, whisk together the lemon juice, olive oil, grated ginger, and thyme. Pour over the halibut, spreading the mixture evenly over the fish.

Bake for 12 to 15 minutes, or until the fish is opaque and flakes when pierced with a fork. The size and thickness of the fish will affect the cooking time.

Serve with the pan juices spooned over the fish. Season generously with pepper and with a pinch of salt, if desired.

NOTE: For a more elegant presentation, put each piece of fish in a small oval baking dish. Top with equal amounts of sauce and bake the fish for 12 to 15 minutes. Serve the fish in the dishes.

NUTRITIONAL ANALYSIS (per serving):

Total carbohydrates: 1 g / Protein: 36 g / Fat: 11 g / Dietary fiber: 0 g / Calories: 260

Baked Salmon with Tomato Salsa

NOTHING BEATS A GOOD SALMON FILLET FOR A RICH, SATISFYING MEAL. We like to buy wild Alaskan salmon because farmed salmon is not as tasty.

SERVES 4

1 tablespoon **OLIVE OIL**

1¹/2 pounds **SALMON FILLETS**

4 large **PLUM TOMATOES**, cored and diced

¹/2 **RED ONION**, chopped

¹/2 **ORANGE BELL PEPPER**, diced

¹/2 bunch **FRESH CILANTRO**, chopped (thick stems removed; about ¹/2 cup)

1 **HOT CHILI PEPPER**, such as a jalapeño or serrano, seeded and diced, optional

1 teaspoon **DRIED OREGANO**

1 large clove **GARLIC**, thinly sliced

JUICE OF 3 LIMES

¹/4 teaspoon **RED PEPPER FLAKES**, optional

3 to 4 tablespoons minced **FLAT-LEAF PARSLEY**, optional

Preheat the oven to 425°F.

Brush the olive oil in a baking pan large enough to hold the salmon fillets comfortably. Lay the salmon in the pan.

In a bowl, combine the tomatoes, onion, bell pepper, cilantro, chili pepper, if using, oregano, and garlic. Add the lime juice and pepper flakes, if using, and toss to mix. You will have about 4 cups. Spoon the salsa and juices around the salmon in the pan, spooning a little on top, too. Cover with aluminum foil.

Bake for 10 to 12 minutes. Remove the foil and check for doneness. If the salmon is not opaque and flakes when prodded with a fork, replace the foil and bake for 8 to 10 minutes longer, or until cooked. Check several times during cooking. Serve immediately, sprinkled with parsley, if desired.

NUTRITIONAL ANALYSIS (per serving):

Total carbohydrates: 10 g / Protein: 40 g / Fat: 16 g / Dietary fiber: 2 g / Calories: 340

My clients and I love the food from the Pump; it's well balanced and free of saturated fat and artificial ingredients. One of my favorite plates after a good workout is the Diesel—it's a great source of protein and fiber. It requires a variety of exercises and balanced nutrition to get maximum results from your workout. I recommend eating food from the Pump restaurants.

—LALO FUENTES
www.LaloFitness.com

Baked Salmon with Cauliflower and Lemon Sauce

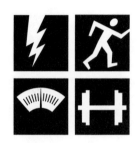

THIS DISH IS A TREAT. The salmon and the cauliflower taste incredible together. Cauliflower adds volume and keeps you satisfied.

SERVES 4

SALMON:

OLIVE OIL COOKING SPRAY

6 ounces **CAULIFLOWER FLORETS**, sliced in half (about 6 florets)

1½ pounds **SALMON FILLETS** or **STEAKS**

2 teaspoons **GRANULATED ONION-PARSLEY MIX**, such as Mrs. Dash

DRESSING:

JUICE FROM 1 LARGE OR 2 MEDIUM LEMONS

¼ cup **WATER**

¼ teaspoon freshly ground **BLACK PEPPER**

10 to 12 large **FRESH BASIL LEAVES**, torn

Preheat the oven to 350°F. Spray a baking pan large enough to hold the salmon in a single layer with cooking spray.

In a pot of boiling water, blanch the cauliflower florets for about 2 minutes until they begin to soften. Drain.

Lay the salmon in the pan. Scatter the cauliflower florets over the salmon and sprinkle with the onion-parsley mix. Spray the cauliflower with a very small amount of cooking spray.

Meanwhile, to make the sauce, squeeze the lemon juice into a cup measure. It should measure approximately ¼ cup. Add an equal amount of water. Stir in the black pepper.

Bake the salmon, uncovered, for 25 to 30 minutes. After about 15 minutes, whisk the lemon mixture and pour over the salmon. Continue to cook until the salmon is cooked through and flakes when prodded with a fork.

Serve with basil leaves sprinkled over the fish for garnish.

NUTRITIONAL ANALYSIS (per serving):
Total carbohydrates: 3 g / Protein: 39 g / Fat: 13 g / Dietary fiber: 1 g / Calories: 290

Fillet of Flounder with Pesto

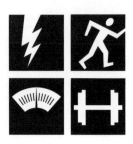

WOW! WE LOVE THIS DISH with a light pesto sauce spread directly on the flounder before it's broiled to a perfect turn. Flounder is mild tasting, making room for the more powerful flavor of the basil and pine nut pesto. When you're finished with your meal, you feel satisfied but never overfed. Instead you will feel pleasingly sated.

SERVES 6

3 tablespoons **PINE NUTS**

2 large bunches **FRESH BASIL**, large stems discarded, leaves washed and shaken dry (leave water clinging to the leaves; about 2 cups loosely packed leaves)

JUICE OF 1 LEMON

2 cloves **GARLIC**, coarsely chopped

1 tablespoon **OLIVE OIL**

Pinch of **SEA SALT**, optional

OLIVE OIL COOKING SPRAY

6 fillets **FLOUNDER** or **SEA BASS** (about 2 pounds)

Spread the pine nuts in a small, dry skillet. Toast over medium heat for 1 to 2 minutes, shaking the pan gently, until the pine nuts are lightly browned and fragrant.

In the bowl of a food processor fitted with the metal blade, combine the basil, lemon juice, garlic, pine nuts, oil, and salt, if using. Process the pesto until nearly smooth but with a little texture.

Preheat the broiler. Spray the broiling pan with cooking spray.

Lay the fillets in a single layer in the pan and spread with the pesto. Broil 5 to 6 inches from the heat for 8 to 10 minutes or until the fish is cooked through, flakes when prodded with a fork, and is opaque.

NUTRITIONAL ANALYSIS (per serving):
Total carbohydrates: 2 g / Protein: 26 g / Fat: 7 g / Dietary fiber: 1 g / Calories: 180

TIPS FOR WHEN YOU VACATION/TRAVEL

· Pack emergency snacks like protein bars, rice cakes, dried fruits, and nuts.

· If you take vitamins and supplements, bring them.

· Be sure that you will have access to fresh vegetables, good salads, and good quality protein.

· When you get to your destination, stop in a market to get water and fruit so that it is always available.

· Make every effort to fit in forty minutes of moderate exercise even when you are away.

· If you drink, stick to red or white wine. Eliminate heavy liquor.

· Be sure to get plenty of rest and sun.

· A massage is great for your muscles.

· Remember, love your body more than you love junk food.

06.
Lean Meat and Poultry

Strip Steak with Mushrooms and Peppers / Rib-Eye Steak with Roasted Garlic / Steak with Thyme and Mustard / Steak Pizzaiola / Grilled Sirloin with Portobello Mushrooms / Flank Steak with Green Peppers and Onion Flakes / Chopped Sirloin with Basil and String Beans / Boneless Leg of Lamb with Roasted Vegetables / Herbed Lamb Chops / Baked Chicken Breast with Stewed Peaches / Chicken with Spinach and Ricotta Cheese / Marinated Garlic-Rosemary Chicken / Baked Chicken with Sun-Dried Tomatoes / Baked Chicken Breast with Lemongrass / Grilled Lemon Chicken / Roast Turkey Breast for Slicing / Tomato-Onion-Red Pepper Ragù

Strip Steak with Mushrooms and Peppers

THIS IS A GOOD EXAMPLE OF HOW TO ENJOY STEAK HEALTHFULLY. It's suggestive of a typical dish of steak with peppers and onions you might eat at a restaurant but without the grease. We toss the vegetables with mushrooms for extra moisture, juiciness, and flavor. The number of veggies with the steak works out to a balanced, tasty meal.

SERVES 4

10 ounces **WHITE** or **CREMINI MUSHROOMS**, sliced (5 to 6 cups)

1/2 large **RED BELL PEPPER**, coarsely chopped

1/2 large **YELLOW ONION**, coarsely chopped

3 tablespoons **BALSAMIC VINEGAR**

1 tablespoon **OLIVE OIL**

1 1/2 to 2 pounds **STRIP STEAK**, about 1 1/2 inches thick

1 tablespoon fresh chopped **ROSEMARY LEAVES**

1 teaspoon freshly ground **BLACK PEPPER**

SEA SALT, optional

Preheat the oven to 350°F.

In a large bowl, toss the mushrooms, pepper, and onion with the vinegar and olive oil. Spread the vegetables in a shallow baking pan and roast for 25 to 30 minutes, depending on how well done you like vegetables.

Use a spatula to scrape the vegetables from the pan. Transfer to a plate and cover with aluminum foil to keep warm.

Meanwhile, preheat the broiler.

Season the steak on both sides with rosemary and pepper. Lay in a broiler pan and broil 5 to 6 inches from the heat for 5 to 7 minutes. Turn and broil for 5 to 6 minutes longer for medium rare, or until done to the degree of doneness desired.

Season the steak with pepper and with salt, if desired.

Let the steak rest for about 5 minutes. Slice and serve topped with the mushroom mixture.

NUTRITIONAL ANALYSIS (per serving):
Total carbohydrates: 7 g / Protein: 33 g / Fat: 23 g / Dietary fiber: 0 g / Calories: 380

Rib-Eye Steak with Roasted Garlic

IT MAY COME AS A PLEASANT SURPRISE TO DISCOVER how mellow and sweet garlic is when it's roasted. Here we spread it over juicy broiled rib-eye steak almost as though it's butter. The garlic gets very hot in the oven, so handle with care. This dish calls for a glass of nice red wine!

SERVES 4

JUICE OF 2 LEMONS
1 tablespoon fresh **THYME**
½ teaspoon freshly ground **BLACK PEPPER**

2 heads **GARLIC**
Four 8-ounce **RIB-EYE STEAKS**

Preheat the oven to 375°F.

In a small bowl, whisk together the lemon juice, thyme, and pepper.

Pull the outer papery skin from the garlic heads but leave a thin skin to hold the cloves together. Lay a large sheet of aluminum foil on the work surface and arrange the heads in the center. Sprinkle 2 tablespoons of the lemon dressing over them. Reserve the rest of the dressing. Wrap the heads securely in the foil and roast for 45 to 50 minutes, or until the garlic pulp is soft. Unwrap and set aside to cool.

Turn off the oven and preheat the broiler.

Lay the steaks on a rack in a broiler pan and drizzle with the remaining lemon dressing. Broil 5 to 6 inches from the heat for 5 minutes, turn, and broil for 4 to 6 minutes longer for medium rare.

Squeeze the garlic pulp from the individual cloves. Put the soft pulp in a bowl and serve it alongside the steaks or spread it over the top of the steaks while they are hot from the broiler.

NUTRITIONAL ANALYSIS (per serving):
Total carbohydrates: 5 g / Protein: 39 g / Fat: 21 g / Dietary fiber: 0 g / Calories: 380

Steak with Thyme and Mustard

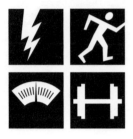

WHEN YOU EAT THIS MUCH PROTEIN—a full-flavored flank steak—with enough vegetables, your body has an easier time absorbing it, which is why we suggest eating this with steamed spinach or broccoli. The mustard and thyme give the steak great flavor without any salt or sauce.
SERVES 4

1½ pounds **FLANK STEAK**

1 tablespoon roughly chopped **THYME LEAVES**

1½ tablespoons **DIJON MUSTARD**

Preheat the broiler. Put a broiler pan in the oven for about 5 minutes to heat it as the broiler heats up.

Remove the pan and lay the steak in it. Sprinkle the thyme over the steak. Broil 5 or 6 inches from the heat for 7 minutes. Turn the steak and broil for 7 to 8 minutes longer for medium-rare meat. Broil the steak longer for better done meat.

Spread the mustard on top of the steak and return it to the oven (not the broiler), which will be hot from the broiler, for 3 to 5 minutes, or until the mustard is warm. Let the steak rest for about 5 minutes before slicing.

NUTRITIONAL ANALYSIS (per serving):
Total carbohydrates: 0 g / Protein: 34 g / Fat: 10 g / Dietary fiber: 0 g / Calories: 240

Steak Pizzaiola

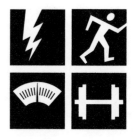

THIS IS A GREAT WAY TO EAT RIB-EYE OR ANY OTHER STEAK: piled high with a delicious, slightly sweet mixture of tomatoes, peppers, and mushrooms that broil alongside the steaks. You will have lots of veggies, and if you don't eat them all, save them for an egg white omelet the next morning. We especially like this dish with a little of our Guacamole the Pump Way (page 14).
SERVES 4

10 ripe **TOMATOES**, cored and coarsely chopped

10 ounces **WHITE** or **CREMINI MUSHROOMS**, sliced (5 to 6 cups)

2 **RED BELL PEPPERS**, seeded and diced

2 tablespoons **DRIED BASIL**

Four 1-inch-thick **RIB-EYE STEAKS**, about 8 ounces each

Preheat the broiler.

In a large saucepan, cook the tomatoes, mushrooms, and peppers over low heat for 4 to 5 minutes, stirring gently, until the vegetables soften and are hot. Do not add water. Stir to prevent sticking. Add the basil, stir to mix, and then remove the pan from the heat. Cover and set aside. You will have about 4 cups of vegetables.

In a dry 12-inch skillet, sear the steaks over high heat for 2 to 3 minutes on each side until brown. Transfer to a broiler pan.

Using a slotted spoon, spoon the tomato-mushroom mixture around the steaks without covering them. Add about 2 cups of the pan juices from the vegetables to the steak, or enough to reach the top of the steaks.

Broil for 4 to 5 minutes for medium rare. Cook longer for better done meat.

Let the steak rest for about 5 minutes and then slice on the diagonal. Serve with the vegetables spooned over it.

NUTRITIONAL ANALYSIS (per serving):
Total carbohydrates: 23 g / Protein: 43 g / Fat: 9 g / Dietary fiber: 3 g / Calories: 480

Grilled Sirloin with Portobello Mushrooms

THIS IS A LOT OF FUN TO PREPARE IN THE SUMMERTIME, when you're doing a lot of grilling. Serving the lean sirloin steak with a savory mixture of mushrooms, onions, and peppers also cooked on the grill raises the satisfaction factor. Perfect with a glass of wine!

SERVES 4

OLIVE OIL COOKING SPRAY

2 to 2¼ pounds **TOP SIRLOIN**, bone in or boneless, any fat trimmed

2 tablespoons chopped fresh **ROSEMARY**

5 tablespoons **BALSAMIC VINEGAR**

1½ tablespoons **DIJON MUSTARD**

½ teaspoon freshly ground **BLACK PEPPER**

Pinch of **SEA SALT,** optional

2 cups sliced **PORTOBELLO MUSHROOMS** (about 5 ounces)

1 small **YELLOW ONION**, chopped

1 **YELLOW BELL PEPPER**, diced

Lightly coat the grilling rack with cooking spray. Prepare a charcoal or gas grill so that the coals are medium hot.

Rub the steak on both sides with the rosemary and set aside.

In a small bowl, whisk together the vinegar, mustard, pepper, and salt, if using.

In a mixing bowl, combine the mushrooms, onion, and pepper. Toss with the balsamic dressing and transfer to a 9-by-13-inch aluminum pan, cover tightly with aluminum foil, and place on the grill. Cook for 15 to 20 minutes, removing the foil and tossing several times.

Push the pan to the side of the grill and lay the steak over the coals. Cook for 15 to 20 minutes for medium-rare meat or until it reaches the desired doneness. Turn it once or twice during grilling.

Slice the meat into diagonal strips and serve with the vegetables.

NUTRITIONAL ANALYSIS (per serving):

Total carbohydrates: 13 g / Protein: 47 g / Fat: 11 g / Dietary fiber: 2 g / Calories: 350

Flank Steak with Green Peppers and Onion Flakes

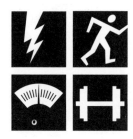

FOR A FAST MEAL, WE LIKE THIS FLANK STEAK. It is delicious with steamed veggies. Spritz the peppers with olive oil spray before you broil them to help them cook evenly without burning.
SERVES 4

1½ to 2 pounds **FLANK STEAK**
2 tablespoons **ONION FLAKES**
1 large **GREEN BELL PEPPER**, seeded and
　chopped into large chunks
OLIVE OIL COOKING SPRAY

　Preheat the broiler.
　Lay the steak in a broiling pan and sprinkle with half the onion flakes. Broil 5 or 6 inches from the flame for 8 minutes.
　Turn the steak over, sprinkle with the remaining onion flakes. Distribute the chunks of pepper around the steak but do not put them on top of it. Spray the pepper lightly with cooking spray. Broil for about 8 minutes longer for medium rare. Cook for longer for better done steak.
　Let the steak rest for about 5 minutes. Slice on the diagonal and serve.

NUTRITIONAL ANALYSIS (per serving):
Total carbohydrates: 3 g / Protein: 34 g / Fat: 11 g / Dietary fiber: 1 g / Calories: 250

Chopped Sirloin with Basil and String Beans

WHEN YOU ARE ESTABLISHING A WORKOUT SCHEDULE, it's essential to eat enough protein, and chopped sirloin is a good source. We serve this with crunchy steamed string beans. With enough protein, you have energy. When you have energy, you have resolve! Steve likes the tomatoes with cumin while Elena prefers them with oregano. Both are delicious.

SERVES 4

2 large **ONIONS**, chopped

2 pounds lean chopped **SIRLOIN**

1/2 bunch fresh **BASIL**, leaves roughly torn

5 **BAY LEAVES**

2 pounds **TOMATOES**, cored and diced (about 5 large tomatoes)

2 teaspoons **CUMIN** or **DRIED OREGANO**

1/2 teaspoon **SALT**, optional

1/2 teaspoon freshly **GROUND PEPPER**, optional

1 pound **STRING BEANS**, trimmed

Heat a large saucepan over medium-low heat. Put the onions in the pan, cover, and cook for 3 to 4 minutes, stirring often to prevent sticking, until softened. Push the onions to the side of the pan.

Add the meat, raise the heat to medium, and cook for 6 to 8 minutes, stirring constantly until there is not much pink remaining.

Pour off and discard accumulated pan juices. Add the basil and bay leaves and cook for about 2 minutes.

Add the tomatoes and cook uncovered for 3 to 5 minutes, stirring, or until they soften and release their juices. Stir in the cumin or oregano and salt and pepper to taste, if using.

Meanwhile, steam the string beans for 3 to 4 minutes in an electric steamer or in a steamer basket set over boiling water, or until crisp-tender.

Put the string beans in a serving dish. Remove the bay leaves from the chopped meat. Spoon the meat over the beans as though you are spooning it over pasta. Serve immediately.

NUTRITIONAL ANALYSIS (per serving):
Total carbohydrates: 3 g / Protein: 34 g / Fat: 11 g / Dietary fiber: 1 g / Calories: 250

Boneless Leg of Lamb with Roasted Vegetables

HERE'S ANOTHER GREAT RECIPE FOR THE GRILL. Boneless leg of lamb—or butterflied leg of lamb, as it's also called—is one of the best meats for cooking outdoors. We marinate the lamb with a lemongrass and sherry marinade and toss the veggies with the same flavors for a tasty treat.

SERVES 8

1/2 cup **DRY SHERRY**

2 large cloves **GARLIC**, minced

One 4-inch-long piece fresh **LEMONGRASS**, halved lengthwise

2 teaspoons dried **THYME**

1 teaspoon dried **OREGANO**

Pinch of **SEA SALT**, optional

Freshly ground **BLACK PEPPER**

41/2- to 5-pound boneless **LEG OF LAMB**

2 **YELLOW ONIONS**, sliced

2 **ZUCCHINI**, ends trimmed and sliced

2 **YELLOW SQUASH**, ends trimmed and sliced

2 tablespoons **OLIVE OIL**

OLIVE OIL COOKING SPRAY

Preheat the oven to 450°F.

In a small bowl, whisk together the sherry, garlic, lemongrass, thyme, and oregano. Season to taste with salt, if using, and pepper.

Lay the leg of lamb in a shallow nonreactive dish or put it in a large plastic bag. Remove 2 tablespoons of the sherry mixture from the bowl and set aside. Pour the remaining sherry mixture over the lamb. Turn the lamb to coat, cover or seal the bag, and refrigerate for at least 2 and up to 6 hours.

Meanwhile, in a large mixing bowl, toss the onions, zucchini, and yellow squash with the olive oil and the remaining 2 tablespoons of the sherry mixture. Set aside.

Prepare a charcoal or gas grill so that the coals are medium hot. Coat the grill rack with cooking spray. Remove the lamb from the marinade. Grill for 30 to 35 minutes, turning once or twice, for medium rare.

After the lamb has been on the grill for about 10 minutes, arrange the vegetables around the outside of the grill. Cook for 20 to 25 minutes, turning with tongs or a spatula 3 to 4 times or until softened.

Let the lamb rest for about 5 minutes before slicing it. Serve it with the grilled vegetables.

NUTRITIONAL ANALYSIS (per serving):
Total carbohydrates: 10 g / Protein: 45 g / Fat: 18 g / Dietary fiber: 1 g / Calories: 420

Herbed Lamb Chops

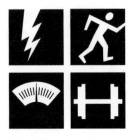

What I like about the Pump food is that it energizes me. Whatever I eat doesn't weigh me down. It sits well in my stomach and satisfies my appetite. The meal gives me the energy to get through my daily routines of work or exercise. We took a week's worth of Pump food to last year's Vermont Mountain Biking Festival. All the other bikers were jealous.

—PAUL SUAREZ

WHEN YOU ARE IN THE MOOD FOR A TREAT, THINK ABOUT LAMB CHOPS! We trim any extra fat and broil them surrounded by onions, which only add sweetness to the already sweet-tasting meat. Doing so does not take much effort, and when you broil the meat instead of sautéing it, it tastes great but you don't need to add extra fat to the pan. A little-known secret about lamb chops: they contain fat-burning L-carnitine.

SERVES 4

2 medium **ONIONS**, chopped, rinsed, and
　drained

OLIVE OIL COOKING SPRAY

Six ¼-inch-thick loin **LAMB CHOPS** (about
　1¾ pounds), fat trimmed

1 tablespoon dried **OREGANO**
Leaves from 2 sprigs fresh **ROSEMARY**,
　coarsely chopped (about 2 tablespoons)

Preheat the broiler.

Put the onions in a bowl and spray lightly with cooking spray. Toss to coat.

Put the lamb chops in the broiler pan and surround them with the onions. Do not put the onions on top of the chops. Sprinkle the oregano and rosemary leaves over the chops and onions.

Broil the chops 5 to 6 inches from the heat for about 7 minutes. Turn and cook for 6 to 7 minutes longer until an instant-read thermometer inserted in the meat without touching the bone registers 140°F for medium-rare meat. Stir the onions when you turn the lamb. For better done lamb, cook a few minutes longer until the meat reaches your desired degree of doneness.

Serve the lamb chops immediately.

NUTRITIONAL ANALYSIS (per serving):
Total carbohydrates: 9 g / Protein: 48 g / Fat: 16 g / Dietary fiber: 2 g / Calories: 380

Baked Chicken Breast with Stewed Peaches

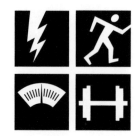

FOR AN EASY, ELEGANT MEAL, PAIR MILD-TASTING CHICKEN WITH FRUIT. The peaches by themselves are amazing (they could double as dessert!) but when cooked with the chicken produce a lovely dish with absolutely no butter or oil. We use crushed almonds where some cooks might use buttered bread crumbs.

SERVES 4

OLIVE OIL

4 boneless, skinless **CHICKEN BREASTS**, 5 to 6 ounces each

SALT, optional

JUICE OF 6 ORANGES (about 3 cups)

4 ripe **PEACHES** (about 1 3/4 pounds), peeled, pitted, and sliced

1/2 cup packed **RAISINS**

1 tablespoon chopped **TOASTED ALMONDS**, for garnish, see Note

Preheat the oven to 350°F. Rub a tiny amount of olive oil in a shallow baking pan large enough to hold the chicken in a single layer.

Lay the breasts in the pan and sprinkle lightly with salt, if desired. Bake for about 35 minutes or until the chicken is cooked through and an instant-read thermometer registers 170°F when inserted in the thickest part of the chicken. Pour off the pan juice from the chicken.

Meanwhile, in a saucepan, combine the orange juice, peaches, and raisins. Bring to a boil, reduce the heat, and simmer, uncovered, for about 20 minutes or until the peaches are soft.

Serve the chicken with the stewed peaches and sauce spooned over it and garnished with almonds.

NOTE: To toast the almonds, put the nuts in a small dry skillet and toast over medium-high heat for 3 to 5 minutes, shaking the pan, until the almonds are fragrant and lightly browned. Remove from the heat and set aside to cool.

NUTRITIONAL ANALYSIS (per serving):
Total carbohydrates: 49 g / Protein: 35 g / Fat: 7 g / Dietary fiber: 1 g / Calories: 390

Chicken with Spinach and Ricotta Cheese

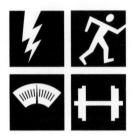

THIS CHICKEN DISH IS AN AMAZING MEAL and a little more complicated than many of our recipes. The extra effort results in flavors that burst in your mouth. We don't use a lot of garlic in our cooking, not liking how it sours our breath, but when you bake garlic, the cloves turn sweet and mellow, rather than sharp and pungent, and so we dare to spread an entire clove on each chicken breast and then pile on the vegetables.

SERVES 6

6 cloves unpeeled **GARLIC**

Two 10-ounce bags fresh **SPINACH**, tough stems removed, rinsed, drained, large leaves torn

8 ounces nonfat **RICOTTA**

2 tablespoons fresh **THYME LEAVES**

¼ teaspoon freshly grated **NUTMEG**

1 teaspoon freshly ground **BLACK PEPPER**

6 boneless, skinless **CHICKEN BREAST** halves, 5 to 6 ounces each

½ pint **GRAPE** or **CHERRY TOMATOES**, stems removed, halved

1 small bunch **SCALLIONS**, trimmed and chopped

Fresh **LEMON JUICE**

SEA SALT, optional

Preheat the oven to 350°F.

Remove only the outer papery skin of the garlic cloves. Wrap in aluminum foil and put on the top rack of the oven. Roast for 50 to 60 minutes or until the cloves are soft. Remove from the oven and set aside, still wrapped loosely in foil to keep warm.

Turn off the oven and preheat the broiler.

Bring a large pot of water to a boil over high heat.

Wash the spinach several times in cool water. The spinach does not have to be dry. Drop the spinach in the boiling water, reduce the heat to medium-high, and cook the spinach for 2 to 3 minutes or until wilted. Alternatively, steam the spinach over boiling water or in an electric steamer. Drain the spinach well.

Transfer the spinach to a large skillet and add the cheese, 2 teaspoons of the thyme, and nutmeg. Cook over medium heat, stirring constantly, for 4 to 5 minutes or until mixed and hot. Season with 1/2 teaspoon of pepper.

Meanwhile, put the chicken breasts on a work surface and cover with plastic wrap or waxed paper. Using a meat mallet or the bottom of a small, heavy frying pan, pound the breasts so that they are about 1/2 inch thick. Sprinkle the chicken on both sides with the remaining thyme and pepper.

Lay the chicken breasts in a broiling pan and broil for 5 to 7 minutes on each side or until cooked through.

Meanwhile, in a medium-size nonstick skillet set over medium heat, cook the tomatoes and scallions, stirring gently, for 2 to 3 minutes or just until heated through and the tomatoes begin to soften.

Arrange the chicken on a platter. Squeeze the softened garlic pulp from each of the cloves over each of the chicken breasts. Spread it thinly over the meat. Top with a heaping scoop of the hot spinach and ricotta mixture. Spoon the tomatoes and scallions over the spinach, season each serving with a squeeze of lemon juice and sea salt, if desired, and serve.

NUTRITIONAL ANALYSIS (per serving):
Total carbohydrates: 18 g / Protein: 39 g / Fat: 3.5 g / Dietary fiber: 5 g / Calories: 250

Marinated Garlic-Rosemary Chicken

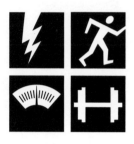

BECAUSE THE CHICKEN IS SOAKED IN A SIMPLE LEMON AND GARLIC MARINADE, this meal is fantastic for planning ahead. The chicken marinates for three hours before it is broiled, and if you prefer, you can grill it over moderately hot coals. We like to serve this with summer squash, steamed zucchini, or cauliflower.

SERVES 4

4 boneless, skinless **CHICKEN BREASTS**, 5 to 6 ounces each

4 cloves **GARLIC**, minced

JUICE AND GRATED ZEST OF 2 LEMONS

3 sprigs fresh **ROSEMARY**

Pinch of **SEA SALT**, optional

In a shallow nonreactive dish, lay the chicken breasts in a single layer. Scatter the garlic over the chicken and then sprinkle with lemon juice and grated zest. Pull the leaves from the rosemary sprigs and sprinkle over the chicken. Add the salt, if using. Turn the meat several times to coat on both sides. Cover with plastic wrap and refrigerate for 3 hours. Turn the chicken once or twice during marinating, if possible.

Preheat the broiler.

Lift the chicken from the marinade and lay in a broiling pan. Spoon the marinade over the chicken. Broil for 8 minutes, turn and cook for 8 to 10 minutes longer, or until the chicken is cooked through and an instant-read thermometer registers 160°F when inserted in the thickest part of the chicken. Serve the chicken immediately.

NUTRITIONAL ANALYSIS (per serving):
Total carbohydrates: 3 g / Protein: 34 g / Fat: 3.5 g / Dietary fiber: 0 g / Calories: 170

Baked Chicken with Sun-dried Tomatoes

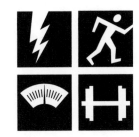

WHEN BAKED WITH THIS HEADY MIXTURE OF SUN-DRIED TOMATOES AND CAPERS, chicken breasts are extremely tasty. You don't need salt and yet the flavor is bright and piquant. Be sure to use oil-packed sun-dried tomatoes; the dry-packed tomatoes are tougher and won't soften as much as they cook.

SERVES 6

3 ounces oil-packed **SUN-DRIED TOMATOES** (about 20 tomatoes), coarsely chopped

3 tablespoons rinsed and drained **CAPERS**

1 tablespoon dried **MARJORAM**

1/4 cup **WHITE BALSAMIC VINEGAR**

2 tablespoons **WATER**

6 boneless, skinless **CHICKEN BREASTS**, each 5 to 6 ounces

OLIVE OIL COOKING SPRAY

Preheat the oven to 425°F.

In a small bowl, combine the tomatoes, capers, and marjoram. Add the vinegar and water and stir to mix.

Lay the chicken on a work surface, cover with plastic wrap, and pound gently with a meat mallet or the flat side of a small, heavy frying pan until about inch thick and even. Put the chicken in a shallow baking pan sprayed with cooking spray that is large enough to hold them in a single layer.

Spoon the tomato mixture over and around the chicken. Bake for 20 to 25 minutes or until the chicken is cooked through and an instant-read thermometer registers 160°F.

Serve the chicken with the sun-dried tomatoes and capers spooned over it.

NUTRITIONAL ANALYSIS (per serving):
Total carbohydrates: 6 g / Protein: 34 g / Fat: 5 g / Dietary fiber: 1 g / Calories: 200

Baked Chicken Breast with Lemongrass

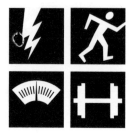

MAKE THIS SOUTHEAST ASIAN–INSPIRED CHICKEN DISH and you will end up with lovely-tasting pan sauce, redolent of lime and orange juice, bold-flavored citrus zest, and the gentle zing of lemongrass. Serve with steamed asparagus, a perfect complement to the citrus flavors of the chicken. **SERVES 6**

3 stalks fresh **LEMONGRASS**, bulb end,
    trimmed and chopped
5 tablespoons fresh **LIME JUICE**
¼ cup fresh **ORANGE JUICE**
¼ teaspoon **CAYENNE PEPPER**

GRATED ZEST OF 1 LIME
GRATED ZEST OF 1 ORANGE
6 boneless, skinless **CHICKEN BREASTS,** each
    5 to 6 ounces
⅓ cup **WATER**

In a shallow nonreactive dish, mix together the lemongrass, lime juice, orange juice, cayenne, lime zest, and orange zest.

Add the chicken to the marinade, turn to coat, cover, and refrigerate for 30 to 60 minutes.

Preheat the oven to 450°F.

Heat a 12-inch ovenproof skillet over medium-high heat.

Lift the chicken from the marinade and reserve the marinade. Stir the water into the marinade and set aside.

Sear the chicken for 2 to 3 minutes on each side or until golden brown. Lower the heat slightly to prevent burning. Add the marinade to the skillet and cook for 1 to 2 minutes longer, stirring to scrape the browned bits from the bottom of the pan and to coat the chicken with the marinade. Transfer to the oven and bake for 15 to 16 minutes, or until an instant-read thermometer registers 160°F.

Serve the chicken with the pan juices.

NUTRITIONAL ANALYSIS (per serving):
Total carbohydrates: 7 g / Protein: 34 g / Fat: 3.5 g / Dietary fiber: 0 g / Calories: 190

Grilled Lemon Chicken

PEOPLE LOVE OUR LEMON CHICKEN. It remains one of the most popular items on our menu. Chicken is a low-fat source of protein, and this recipe makes chicken as delicious as it is healthful. It goes well with steamed vegetables, salads, or brown rice.

SERVES 6

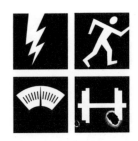

⅓ cup fresh **LEMON JUICE**

1 cup **WATER**

3 teaspoons **DRIED OREGANO**

6 boneless, skinless **CHICKEN BREASTS**, 5 to 6 ounces each

1 large **LEMON**, cut into 12 thin slices

In a large nonreactive bowl, stir together the lemon juice, water, and oregano. Add the chicken breasts, turn to coat, cover, and refrigerate for up to 6 hours.

Light the grill or preheat the broiler.

Lift the chicken from the marinade and let the marinade drip off the meat. Lay the chicken breasts on the grill or in a broiling pan and cook for 5 to 7 minutes on each side or until cooked through.

Serve each chicken breast with 2 slices of lemon.

NUTRITIONAL ANALYSIS (per serving):

Total carbohydrates: 4 g / Protein: 33 g / Fat: 3.5 g / Dietary fiber: 0 g / Calories: 170

Roast Turkey Breast for Slicing

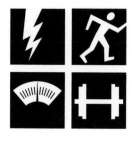

A SIMPLE ROASTED TURKEY BREAST IS GREAT FOR FAMILIES. After the first meal of hot roasted white meat turkey, the breast can be refrigerated and then sliced for sandwiches, salads, and omelets. We like turkey served with brown rice and steamed vegetables. Or serve it alongside a cup of soup. Sliced turkey is a good source of protein and doesn't have much fat. It's best to buy fresh turkey breast, but we know it's far easier to find it frozen in the supermarket. Frozen birds need to defrost (see the note at the end of the recipe), which takes time but isn't difficult.

SERVES 8

One 5½- to 6-pound bone-in **TURKEY BREAST**

3 **CARROTS**, peeled and halved

2 ribs **CELERY**, trimmed and quartered

1 large **ONION**, peeled and cut into wedges

6 to 8 fresh **SAGE LEAVES** or 1 tablespoon dried **SAGE**

6 stems fresh **THYME** (each about 4 inches long)

2 stems fresh **ROSEMARY** (each about 4 inches long)

½ **LEMON**

1 tablespoon **OLIVE OIL**, optional

1 teaspoon **SEA SALT**, optional

½ teaspoon freshly ground **BLACK PEPPER**, optional

1 cup **WATER**

Preheat the oven to 325°F.

Rinse the turkey breast with water. Put on a rack in a roasting pan. Surround the turkey with the carrots, celery, and onion quarters and tuck the herbs in the vegetables and under the turkey. Squeeze the lemon juice over the turkey and tuck the squeezed lemon half under the turkey.

Rub the olive oil over the turkey breast, if using, and season with salt and pepper, if desired. Pour the water around the turkey.

Loosely tent the turkey with aluminum foil and roast for 2 hours. Remove the foil and roast for about 30 minutes longer, or until the skin is crisp and browned, the juices run clear, and an instant-read thermometer inserted in the thickest part of the breast meat registers 170°F. Turkey breast should be cooked for 20 to 25 minutes to the pound.

Lift the breast from the pan and let it rest on a cutting board for about 10 minutes. Discard the vegetables. Slice and serve the turkey.

NOTE: If the turkey breast is frozen, let it defrost in the refrigerator for 24 to 48 hours. You may also defrost it in a sink filled with cold water. Leave the turkey in its wrapping and submerge it in the water. Depending on the size of the breast, this will take from 4 to 8 hours. Never leave it on the countertop to thaw.

VARIATION: Sliced Turkey Breast with Soy Sauce: Lay sliced, cooked turkey in a broiler pan and sprinkle lightly with low-sodium soy sauce. Broil for 8 to 10 minutes, turning the turkey slices once, just until heated through.

NUTRITIONAL ANALYSIS (per serving):
Total carbohydrates: 12 g / Protein: 68 g / Fat: 3 g / Dietary fiber: 5 g / Calories: 360

Tomato-Onion-Red Pepper Ragù

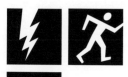

THIS RAGÙ IS ONE OF THE BEST WAYS WE KNOW TO DRESS UP broiled chicken or fish, and it's equally good spooned over salad greens or brown rice, or on a sandwich or burger. It looks pretty and has a pleasing amount of spiciness without being truly hot.

MAKES ABOUT 4 CUPS

1 tablespoon **OLIVE OIL**
3/4 pound diced **YELLOW ONIONS** (about 2½ cups)
1 **RED BELL PEPPER**, diced
2 pints **GRAPE** or **CHERRY TOMATOES**, halved
1/3 cup **WATER** or **RED WINE**
1 teaspoon dried **BASIL**

1 teaspoon minced fresh **ROSEMARY LEAVES**
1/4 teaspoon **RED PEPPER FLAKES**, optional
SEA SALT, optional
Freshly ground **BLACK PEPPER**, optional
1/3 to 1/2 cup torn fresh **BASIL LEAVES**

In a large saucepan or deep sauté pan, heat the olive oil over medium heat. Add the onions, reduce the heat to medium low, cover, and cook for about 5 minutes, stirring occasionally, until softened. Add the pepper and cook, stirring, for about 2 minutes longer until softened. Add the tomatoes, water or wine, basil, and rosemary. Season to taste with pepper flakes, salt, and pepper, if desired.

Cover and cook over medium heat for about 15 minutes until the vegetables soften and the ragù is chunky and thickened.

Just before serving, stir the fresh basil leaves into the ragù. Serve hot, spooned over broiled chicken or fish.

NUTRITIONAL ANALYSIS (per 2-tablespoon serving):
Total carbohydrates: 2 g / Protein: 0 g / Fat: .5 g / Dietary fiber: 1 g / Calories: 15

It is very difficult for me to have to choose one favorite item from the Pump menu as I have so many different dishes that I love when I go in on different days, but if I must, then I would have to say #48, Thunder. The grilled chicken breast with onions, tomatoes, peppers, and low-sodium tomato sauce served over brown rice is excellent! The Pump is an ideal complement whether I or my clients are looking to lose weight, gain muscle mass, eat vegetarian, semi-vegetarian, or non-vegetarian food. You can order dishes either high in carbs or high in protein and all are low in fat, sugar, and sodium, for whatever fitness goal one is looking to obtain. Good nutrition, like exercise, results in countless benefits both physically and psychologically and I would also be so bold to say spiritually as well.

— ALAN BARON, owner/fitness trainer, Prism Fitness

07.
Vegetarian Main Courses

Baked Tofu / Vegetarian Chili / Quinoa with Vegetables / Chickpea Stew with Basil / Kidney Bean and Butternut Squash Stew / Asian Peanut Stir-Fry / Ginger-Tofu Stir-Fry

Baked Tofu

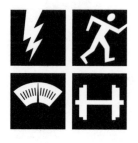

MOST VEGETARIANS LOVE BAKED TOFU, but you don't have to be vegetarian to appreciate its meaty characteristics and the fact that it's a terrific source of protein. We like to put it on top of steamed vegetables or on a salad and add our Carrot-Ginger Dressing or Tahini Dressing.
SERVES 4

2/3 cup **WATER**
1/3 cup reduced-sodium **SOY SAUCE**
2 tablespoons fresh **LIME JUICE**
1 teaspoon toasted **SESAME OIL**
1/4 teaspoon **HOT CHILI OIL**, optional
One 1-inch piece fresh **GINGER**, peeled and
    cut into thin slices

2 to 3 **SCALLIONS**, white and green parts,
    trimmed and cut into 1-inch lengths
14 to 16 ounces **EXTRA-FIRM TOFU**, sliced
    into 8 even slices

Preheat the oven to 375°F.

In a small bowl, whisk together the water, soy sauce, lime juice, sesame oil, and chili oil, if using. Add the ginger and scallions and stir to mix.

Lay the tofu slices in a single layer in an ovenproof glass or ceramic dish measuring about 7 1/2 by 11 1/2 inches. Pour the marinade over the tofu, lifting the slices carefully so that marinade seeps under them and coats both sides of the tofu.

Bake for 25 minutes. Pull the pan from the oven and baste the tofu with the pan juices. Continue baking for 20 to 25 minutes longer or until nearly all the marinade has evaporated. The outside of the tofu will be firm and dark, mahogany brown. The tofu will be creamy white on the inside.

Remove the pan from the oven and baste the tofu again with any liquid remaining in the pan. Using a spatula, carefully lift the tofu from the pan and serve warm. Discard any marinade remaining in the pan.

NUTRITIONAL ANALYSIS (per serving):
Total carbohydrates: 4 g / Protein: 12 g / Fat: 8 g / Dietary fiber: 2 g / Calories: 130

Vegetarian Chili

OUR CUSTOMERS LOVE THIS HEALTHFUL VEGETARIAN CHILI made with three kinds of beans and lots of good-tasting vegetables. Anyway you dish it up, this chili is a grand slam.

SERVES 6

8 **PLUM TOMATOES** (about 2¼ pounds), seeded and diced

4 ribs **CELERY**, diced

5 to 6 **CARROTS**, peeled and diced

3 to 4 large **ONIONS**, diced

2 medium-size **GREEN BELL PEPPERS**, diced

3 **BAY LEAVES**

3½ cups **WATER**

2 cups **THE PUMP'S HOMEMADE TOMATO SAUCE** , page 110

1 cup cooked **RED BEANS**, see Note

1 cup cooked **WHITE KIDNEY BEANS**, see Note

1 cup cooked **BLACK BEANS**, see Note

3 tablespoons **CHILI POWDER**

2 teaspoons **CORIANDER SEEDS**

2 teaspoons **CUMIN**

2 teaspoons **PAPRIKA**

½ teaspoon freshly ground **BLACK PEPPER**

¼ teaspoon **CAYENNE PEPPER**

In large, heavy pot, cook the tomatoes, celery, carrots, onions, peppers, bay leaves, and 1 cup of the water over low heat, covered, for about 20 minutes or until they begin to soften, stirring often to keep from sticking.

Add the remaining 2½ cups of water and bring to a boil over medium-high heat. Reduce the heat to medium and simmer for 20 minutes or until the vegetables are soft, stirring often.

Put the tomato sauce, beans, chili powder, coriander seeds, cumin, paprika, and pepper in the pot and stir well. Cook over medium-low heat for about 1 hour and 15 minutes to give the flavors time to develop and until thickened. Serve immediately.

NOTE: For directions on cooking dried beans, see the box on page 107.

NUTRITIONAL ANALYSIS (per serving):
Total carbohydrates: 49 g / Protein: 12 g / Fat: 3.5 g / Dietary fiber: 14 g / Calories: 260

Quinoa with Vegetables

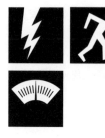

WE PUT NUTRITIOUS QUINOA (PRONOUNCED "KEEN-WA") IN THE SAME CATEGORY AS brown rice and sweet potatoes. It's a terrific complex carbohydrate and the only grain with all the essential amino acids. Although higher in protein than others, this grain still does not have enough for your daily needs, but this dish is good to eat on a day when you have overloaded on protein at other meals. This ancient grain originated in the Andes but is now grown in Colorado and other high-altitude places. It cooks more quickly than rice and blends nicely with softened vegetables. We suggest sweet onions and tomatoes, but you could just as easily serve it with other vegetables.
SERVES 4

1 small **VIDALIA ONION**, chopped
1 large **TOMATO**, cored and chopped
1 rib **CELERY**, finely chopped
2 large **BAY LEAVES**

4 cups **WATER**
2 cups **QUINOA**
¼ cup chopped **FLAT-LEAF PARSLEY**

In a heavy pot set over low heat, cook the onion, tomato, celery, and bay leaves, partially covered, for 10 to 12 minutes or until soft, stirring occasionally to prevent sticking.

Meanwhile, in a large pot, bring the water to a boil over medium-high heat. Stir in the quinoa, then reduce the heat to medium so the water is simmering. Cover and cook for about 12 minutes or until nearly soft.

Remove the quinoa from the heat, stir in the softened vegetables and parsley (remove and discard the bay leaves), and set aside, covered, for about 10 minutes until the flavors meld. Serve immediately.

NUTRITIONAL ANALYSIS (per serving):
Total carbohydrates: 63 g / Protein: 12 g / Fat: 5 g / Dietary fiber: 6 g / Calories: 340

Chickpea Stew with Basil

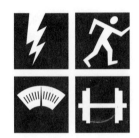

STEVE IS FOND OF CHICKPEAS FOR A NUMBER OF REASONS, not the least of which is because, when he was a child growing up in Greece, his mother cooked them often. We find them filling and satisfying, and this easy stew is a whole meal. Let's face it, whenever you combine tomatoes with basil you have good flavor.

SERVES 6

2 large **VIDALIA ONIONS**, chopped

1/3 cup **WATER**

6 plum **TOMATOES**, diced

4 cups **WATER**

1/3 cup **OLIVE OIL**

2 tablespoons finely minced **FRESH
	LEMONGRASS** cut from the bulb (root)
	end of the stalk

4 cups cooked **CHICKPEAS**, page 107

10 fresh **BASIL LEAVES**, chopped, for garnish

1 tablespoon fresh **LEMON JUICE**

1/4 teaspoon **SALT**, optional

RED PEPPER FLAKES

In a heavy saucepan, cook the onions and water over low heat for 10 to 12 minutes until softened, stirring occasionally to prevent sticking. Add the tomatoes, cover, and cook for 15 minutes or until very soft.

Meanwhile, bring the water, oil, and lemongrass to a boil over medium-high heat. Add the softened vegetables and the chickpeas. Immediately reduce the heat to medium-low. Mix well. Cover and simmer gently for 20 to 30 minutes, stirring occasionally, until the flavors meld.

Gently stir the basil, lemon juice, and salt, if using, into the stew. Sprinkle with red pepper flakes, and serve.

NUTRITIONAL ANALYSIS (per serving):
Total carbohydrates: 39 g / Protein: 11 g / Fat: 15 g / Dietary fiber: 10 g / Calories: 330

Kidney Bean and Butternut Squash Stew

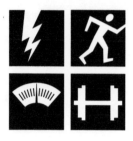

THIS STEW IS IDEAL FOR ANYONE TRYING TO SHED A FEW POUNDS. It's filling and hearty and good enough to eat day after day. Serve it with a salad for a great meal. For extra protein, add a can of tuna or some grilled chicken. The butternut squash is sweet and thickens the stew without the addition of cream or flour. The sun-dried tomatoes cut easily with kitchen shears, if you have them. **SERVES 6**

1 large **YELLOW ONION**, chopped

2 cups **VEGETABLE STOCK** or **WATER**

1 **BUTTERNUT SQUASH**, peeled, seeded, and cut into approximately 1-inch chunks

2 cups (6 ounces) sliced **CREMINI** or **WHITE MUSHROOMS**

2 cups cooked **RED KIDNEY BEANS,** page 107

20 dry-packed **SUN-DRIED TOMATOES**, coarsely chopped

1 1/2 tablespoons drained and rinsed **CAPERS**

2 tablespoons extra-virgin **OLIVE OIL**

1/4 tablespoon **SEA SALT**, optional

1/3 cup chopped **FLAT-LEAF PARSLEY**, optional

In a heavy saucepan, cook the onion and 1/4 cup of the stock or water over low heat for 10 to 12 minutes until softened, stirring occasionally to prevent sticking. Add the squash chunks, mushrooms, and 1 cup of the stock or water, raise the heat to medium, cover the pan, and cook for 12 to 15 minutes or until very soft.

Add the remaining stock or water, kidney beans, sun-dried tomatoes, capers, olive oil, and salt, if using, and stir well to mix. Reduce the heat to low and cook for 12 to 15 minutes or until the flavors blend. Serve immediately garnished with parsley.

NUTRITIONAL ANALYSIS (per serving):
Total carbohydrates: 39 g / Protein: 9 g / Fat: 7 g / Dietary fiber: 3 g / Calories: 230

I have been involved in fitness for over 15 years now and I have eaten at the Pump since it opened. The owners take great care in making sure they maintain the healthiest food with the best flavor. Who says that healthy food has to be bland? In a world with unhealthy alternatives all around us, it's fortunate to have a restaurant like the Pump.

—GLENN BROWN, personal fitness trainer

Asian Peanut Stir-Fry

We always have a lot of fun when we make this stir-fry. Since it includes peanuts and peanut butter, it has intense flavor. The bok choy bulks up the dish and the tofu provides protein. We make it with soy sauce, but low-sodium wheat-free tamari is a great alternative. Elena's mother, a confirmed vegetarian, loves this dish! Serve it with Green Cabbage Salad on page 49 instead of rice.

SERVES 6

I eat [at the Pump] every day I'm at work, and sometimes twice a day. Pasta can be substituted for rice (which I can eat), nothing is cooked with butter, nothing is fried, the chicken is lean, and everything's fresh and healthy. My allergies don't suffer and my taste buds are happy. Almost all of my coworkers order out from the Pump as well. For us, it's not just takeout; it's a religion. If the Pump ever becomes a publicly traded company, I'll be the first to buy stock.

—JOSH TARJAN, customer

3 tablespoons **OLIVE OIL**

3 ribs **CELERY**, cut into medium dice (about 2 cups)

10 ounces **SHIITAKE MUSHROOMS**, trimmed and sliced (about 3 cups)

1 medium **YELLOW ONION**, chopped

8 to 10 **SCALLIONS**, white and green parts, sliced (about 1½ cups)

1 small head **BOK CHOY**, sliced

1 large **RED BELL PEPPER**, seeded and chopped

4 cloves **GARLIC**, sliced

6 tablespoons low-sodium **SOY SAUCE**

4 tablespoons smooth reduced-fat **PEANUT BUTTER**

1 pound **FIRM TOFU**, drained well, cut into ½-inch cubes (about 3 cups)

2 tablespoons **PEANUTS**, chopped, for garnish

Heat the olive oil in a large skillet or wok over medium-high heat. Add the celery, mushrooms, onion, scallions, bok choy, red pepper, and garlic, toss to mix, and cook for 3 to 5 minutes, or until the vegetables begin to soften. You may need to cook this in two batches.

Add the soy sauce and peanut butter and stir for about 1 minute or until the peanut butter liquefies.

Stir in the tofu and cook for 1 to 2 minutes, stirring, until the tofu is heated through.

Transfer to a serving dish and garnish with chopped peanuts.

NUTRITIONAL ANALYSIS (per serving):

Total carbohydrates: 21 g / Protein: 15 g / Fat: 18 g / Dietary fiber: 5 g / Calories: 290

Ginger-Tofu Stir-Fry

THE VEGETABLES IN THIS TOFU STIR-FRY, flavored with fresh ginger and toasted sesame oil, make it robust and satisfying. A little ginger goes a long way in terms of flavor. Serve it with brown rice or quinoa, if you like, or eat it on its own. We sometimes sprinkle a little brown rice over the stir-fry before we eat it, which we find quells any craving we might have for carbohydrates without overeating them.

SERVES 4

3 tablespoons **WHITE WINE** or **RICE WINE VINEGAR**

2 tablespoons toasted **SESAME OIL**

2 tablespoons low-sodium **SOY SAUCE**

2 tablespoons shredded fresh **GINGER**

1 small **LEEK**, trimmed, split lengthwise, washed, sliced crosswise (about 2/3 cup)

1/2 large **RED BELL PEPPER**, seeded and cut into 2-inch-long matchsticks

14 ounces **FIRM TOFU**, diced

2 medium **CARROTS**, peeled and coarsely shredded

2 small **ZUCCHINI**, cut into 2-inch-long matchsticks

8 ounces **SNOW PEAS**, trimmed (about 2 cups)

1/4 cup chopped fresh **CILANTRO**, optional

RED PEPPER FLAKES, optional

In a wok, whisk together the vinegar, sesame oil, soy sauce, and ginger. Set over medium-high heat and when hot, add the leek and pepper and stir-fry for 1 or 2 minutes or until the vegetables begin to soften.

Add the tofu, carrots, zucchini, and snow peas and cook for 4 to 6 minutes or until the vegetables are crisp-tender and the tofu is heated through. Serve garnished with cilantro and red pepper flakes, if desired.

NUTRITIONAL ANALYSIS (per serving):
Total carbohydrates: 15 g / Protein: 14 g / Fat: 14 g / Dietary fiber: 4 g / Calories: 230

COOKING BLACK-EYED PEAS

In a large bowl or pot, soak 1 pound of black-eyed or yellow peas in cold water to cover by three or four inches. Soak for 30 minutes. Drain in a colander and rinse well with cool, running water.

Put the peas in a large pot and add water. The water should fill the pot to four times the depth of the peas.

Bring to a boil over high heat, uncovered. Remove any foam that rises to the surface of the pot. Reduce the heat and simmer for about 30 minutes, or until tender but not mushy.

Drain in a colander and rinse well with cold water, until cool. Drain and use in a recipe. You will have about 7 cups of cooked peas.

COOKING DRIED BEANS

In a large bowl, soak 1 pound of dried beans (red, white, or black) in cold water to cover by three or four inches. Soak for 24 hours. Drain in a colander and rinse well with cool, running water.

Put the beans in a large pot and add water. The water should fill the pot to four times the depth of the beans.

Bring to a boil over high heat, uncovered. Remove any foam that rises to the surface of the pot. Reduce the heat and simmer for the suggested amount of time, or until tender but not mushy.

Red kidney beans: 1 to $1^1/_2$ hours

White chickpeas: $1^1/_2$ to 2 hours

White navy beans: $1^1/_2$ to 2 hours

White Great Northern beans: 1 to $1^1/_2$ hours

Black beans: 30 to 60 minutes

Drain in a colander and rinse well with cold water, until cool. Drain and use in a recipe. You will have about 6 cups of cooked beans.

08.
Pizza and Burgers

The Pump's Homemade Tomato Sauce / Whole Wheat Tomato Pizza / Steak-and-Onion Pizza / Chicken-Spinach Pizza / Turkey Burger Pizza / Tofu Pizza / Nature Burger and Tomato Pizza / Nature Burger / Rookie Steak Burger / Pizza-Style Turkey Burger

The Pump's Homemade Tomato Sauce

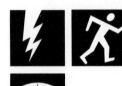

WE MAKE THIS SAUCE ALL THE TIME—it's light, tasty, versatile, and easy to make. There is not much sodium, so you never feel thirsty after eating this spread on pizza. It keeps in the refrigerator for up to three days; we don't recommend freezing it.

MAKES ABOUT 1 1/3 CUPS

1 small **ONION**, quartered

1 clove **GARLIC**, optional

6 **PLUM TOMATOES**, cored, seeded, and
    quartered

2 teaspoons **OLIVE OIL**

1/2 teaspoon dried **OREGANO**

1/2 teaspoon dried **BASIL**

SEA SALT, optional

In the bowl of a food processor fitted with the metal blade, chop onion and garlic by pulsing 2 or 3 times. Add the tomatoes and pulse 4 to 5 times. The mixture should have some texture. Alternately, chop the tomatoes, onions, and garlic into small pieces.

In a medium saucepan, heat the oil and add the tomato-onion mixture. Cook over medium-low heat, stirring to prevent sticking, for about 5 minutes until heated through and bubbling.

Add the oregano and basil. Cook, uncovered, for about 20 minutes, stirring frequently, until thickened to a sauce-like consistency and most of the liquid evaporates. Taste and season with salt, if desired.

NUTRITIONAL ANALYSIS (per 2-tablespoon serving):
Total carbohydrates: 3 g / Protein: 0 g / Fat: 1 g / Dietary fiber: 1 g / Calories: 20

Whole Wheat Tomato Pizza

EVERYONE WHO LIKES PIZZA GETS A CRAVING NOW AND THEN for the tomato-and-cheese-topped pie. This simple pizza will quell those cravings. We top this and many of our other pizzas with nonfat mozzarella, but you can substitute low-fat mozzarella or soy cheese, if you prefer. Eating this pizza—or any in this chapter—will leave you feeling great and very satisfied!

SERVES 4

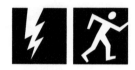

4 whole wheat 7-inch **PITA BREADS**

1⅓ cups **THE PUMP'S HOMEMADE TOMATO SAUCE**, page 110

12 ounces nonfat **MOZZARELLA**, shredded (about 3 cups)

Preheat the oven to 425°F.

Put the pitas on the oven rack and toast for 4 to 5 minutes until lightly crisped. Take care they do not burn. Remove from the oven.

Lay the pitas on a baking sheet. Spoon ⅓ cup of tomato sauce over each pita and top each with an equal amount of cheese.

Bake for about 6 minutes or until the cheese melts. Serve immediately.

NUTRITIONAL ANALYSIS (per serving):
Total carbohydrates: 43 g / Protein: 34 g / Fat: 3 g / Dietary fiber: 7 g / Calories: 330

Steak-and-Onion Pizza

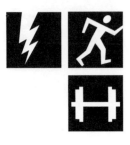

WHEN YOU'RE IN THE MOOD FOR A SUBSTANTIAL PIZZA, this pizza is the ticket. We use lean sirloin, which you can buy on or off the bone; either way, the flavor is good. This pizza is a meal in itself, especially if you pair it with a big salad. What a treat!

SERVES 4

4 large whole wheat 7-inch **PITA BREADS**
1 pound boneless **SIRLOIN STEAK**, cubed
Freshly ground **BLACK PEPPER**
1 small **GREEN BELL PEPPER**, seeded and diced
1 medium **ONION**, cut into strips

¼ cup **WATER**
1⅓ cups **THE PUMP'S HOMEMADE TOMATO SAUCE**, page 110
12 ounces nonfat **MOZZARELLA**, shredded (about 4 cups)

Preheat the oven to 425°F.

Put the pitas on the oven rack and toast for 4 to 5 minutes until lightly crisped. Take care they do not burn. Remove from the oven.

Meanwhile, season the steak with the pepper. In a large nonstick skillet, cook the steak for 2 to 3 minutes over medium-high heat. Remove from the pan and set aside. Pour any fat from the pan.

Put the pepper, onion, and water in the pan, reduce the heat to medium, and cook, uncovered, for 3 to 4 minutes, stirring, until the vegetables begin to soften and the excess liquid reduces almost completely.

Lay the pitas on a baking sheet. Spoon ⅓ cup of tomato sauce over each pita and top each with an equal amount of the steak and vegetables and then with cheese.

Bake for about 6 minutes or until the cheese melts. Serve immediately.

NUTRITIONAL ANALYSIS (per serving):
Total carbohydrates: 46 g / Protein: 56 g / Fat: 8 g / Dietary fiber: 8 g / Calories: 480

Chicken-Spinach Pizza

JUST AS OUR CHICKEN AND SPINACH SANDWICH (page 32) is wildly popular with the Pump's customers, so is this pizza. Same winning flavor combination but a little lighter.
SERVES 4

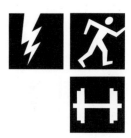

4 large whole wheat 7-inch **PITA BREADS**

20 ounces boneless, skinless **CHICKEN BREAST** meat, cut into small pieces or thin strips

1 large **TOMATO**, cored, diced, and patted dry

½ cup torn fresh **BASIL LEAVES**

1 small clove **GARLIC**, minced, optional

1⅓ cups **THE PUMP'S HOMEMADE TOMATO SAUCE**, page 110

4 ounces fresh **BABY SPINACH LEAVES**, washed, dried, and roughly chopped (about 4 cups)

12 ounces nonfat **MOZZARELLA**, shredded (about 3 cups)

RED PEPPER FLAKES, for sprinkling, optional

Preheat the oven to 425°F.

Put the pitas on the oven rack and toast for 4 to 5 minutes until lightly crisped. Take care they do not burn. Remove from the oven.

Meanwhile, in a large nonstick skillet, cook the chicken for 2 to 3 minutes over medium-high heat, stirring, until browned. Add the tomato, basil, and garlic, if using. Reduce the heat to medium, and cook for 3 to 5 minutes, stirring, until the tomato begins to soften and some of the liquid is reduced. You will have about 4 cups of the chicken-vegetable mixture.

Lay the pitas on the baking sheet. Spoon ⅓ cup of the tomato sauce over each pita and top each with a handful of spinach. Spread the chicken and tomatoes over the spinach and top with cheese.

Bake for about 6 minutes or until the cheese melts and the spinach wilts. Sprinkle with red pepper flakes, if desired, and serve immediately.

NUTRITIONAL ANALYSIS (per serving):
Total carbohydrates: 49 g / Protein: 69 g / Fat: 7 g / Dietary fiber: 10 g / Calories: 520

Turkey Burger Pizza

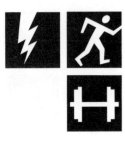

USING GROUND TURKEY TO TOP THE PIZZA GIVES IT AN INTENSITY not found in some of our other pizzas. The turkey, while lean and light, provides a hint of a sausage taste and texture to the pizza for a terrific meal.

SERVES 4

4 large whole wheat 7-inch **PITA BREADS**
1 pound ground **TURKEY BREAST**
1 medium **ONION**, chopped
1½ teaspoons crumbled dried **SAGE**

1⅓ cups **THE PUMP'S HOMEMADE TOMATO SAUCE**, page 110
12 ounces nonfat **MOZZARELLA**, shredded (about 3 cups)

Preheat the oven to 425°F.

Put the pitas on the oven rack and toast for 4 to 5 minutes until lightly crisped. Take care they do not burn. Remove from the oven.

Meanwhile, in a large nonstick skillet, cook the ground turkey 2 to 3 minutes over medium-high heat, stirring, until browned. With a slotted spoon, remove the turkey from the pan and set aside.

Add the onion and sage, reduce the heat to medium, and cook for 1 to 2 minutes, stirring, until the onion begins to soften. Return the turkey to the pan and stir to mix.

Lay the pitas on the baking sheet. Spoon tomato sauce over the pitas and top each with the turkey mixture. Top with cheese and a little more tomato sauce.

Bake for about 6 minutes or until the cheese melts. Serve immediately.

NUTRITIONAL ANALYSIS (per serving):
Total carbohydrates: 46 g / Protein: 69 g / Fat: 4.5 g / Dietary fiber: 8 g / Calories: 500

Tofu Pizza

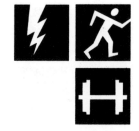

ALTHOUGH WE ARE FAR FROM BEING VEGETARIANS, we love tofu and turn to it time and again as a source of protein. It works well with vegetables, and when veggies and tofu top a pita pizza, the result is incredible.

SERVES 4

3 ounces **BROCCOLI** florets (about 1/3 cup)

1 medium **ONION**, sliced

1 small **GREEN BELL PEPPER**, seeded and sliced

4 whole wheat 7-inch **PITA BREADS**

1 1/3 cups **THE PUMP'S HOMEMADE TOMATO SAUCE**, page 110

2 medium **TOMATOES**, cored, diced, and patted dry

8 ounces **FIRM TOFU**, sliced 1/4 to 1/2 inch thick

12 ounces nonfat **MOZZARELLA**, shredded (about 3 cups)

In a steamer basket set over simmering water or in an electric steamer, steam the broccoli, onion, and pepper for 1 to 2 minutes or until fork-tender. Drain well and set aside.

Preheat the oven to 425°F.

Put the pitas on the oven rack and toast for 4 to 5 minutes until lightly crisped. Take care they do not burn. Remove from the oven.

Lay the pitas on the baking sheet. Spoon 1/3 cup of tomato sauce over each pita and top each with the steamed vegetables and diced tomatoes. Top with slices of tofu and the cheese.

Bake for about 6 minutes or until the cheese melts and the tofu is heated through. Serve immediately.

VARIATION: For a lighter veggie pizza, omit the tofu.

NUTRITIONAL ANALYSIS (per serving):
Total carbohydrates: 52 g / Protein: 42 g / Fat: 8 g / Dietary fiber: 10 g / Calories: 430

Nature Burger and Tomato Pizza

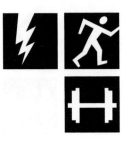

BECAUSE WE ARE SO FOND OF OUR NATURE BURGERS and love pita bread pizzas, we adore this pizza and think it tastes much better than pizzas made with gobs of melted cheese and pepperoni and salami. If you're vegan, use soy cheese instead.

SERVES 4

4 whole wheat 7-inch **PITA BREADS**
4 uncooked **NATURE BURGERS**, page 117
1 1/3 cups **THE PUMP'S HOMEMADE TOMATO SAUCE**, page 110

12 ounces nonfat **MOZZARELLA**, shredded (about 3 cups)

Preheat the oven to 425°F.

Put the pitas on the oven rack and toast for 4 to 5 minutes until lightly crisped. Take care they do not burn. Remove from the oven.

Meanwhile, in a nonstick skillet, cook the burgers over medium-high heat, breaking them up with a fork as they cook, until browned and slightly crispy.

Lay the pitas on a baking sheet. Spoon 1/3 cup of tomato sauce over each pita and top each with an equal amount of browned burger mixture and cheese.

Bake for 6 to 8 minutes or until the cheese melts. Serve immediately.

NUTRITIONAL ANALYSIS (per serving):
Total carbohydrates: 70 g / Protein: 44 g / Fat: 12 g / Dietary fiber: 14 g / Calories: 540

Nature Burger

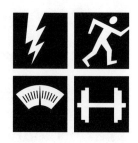

WE LOVE NATURE BURGERS IN PITA BREAD, over salad greens, with brown rice, and even on pizza (see our recipe for the Nature Burger and Tomato Pizza on page 116). These burgers are not similar to the typical nature burger you might buy in a health food store, but have more character and flavor because we are not trying to imitate meat. These are uniquely delicious in and of themselves.

SERVES 4

1 cup cooked **BROWN RICE**, page 139

1 cup cooked **LENTILS**

¼ cup **SUNFLOWER SEEDS**

¾ cup roughly chopped **ONION**

1 tablespoon **BROWN RICE MISO**

1 tablespoon **TAHINI**

¼ cup packed **FLAT-LEAF PARSLEY LEAVES**

¼ cup packed fresh **CELERY LEAVES**

½ teaspoon freshly ground **WHITE PEPPER**

OLIVE OIL COOKING SPRAY

Preheat the oven to 400°F.

In the bowl of a food processor fitted with the metal blade, process the rice, lentils, sunflower seeds, onion, miso, tahini, parsley, celery leaves, and pepper for about 30 seconds. Scrape down the sides and process until well mixed and cohesive. Transfer the mixture to a bowl. You will have about 2¼ cups.

Spray a shallow baking tray with olive oil spray. Put the pan in the oven for about 5 minutes to heat it.

Form the rice mixture into 4 patties and put on the hot pan. Lightly spray the tops of the patties with olive oil spray. Bake for 10 minutes, turn, and lightly spray the patties with more olive oil spray. Bake for 6 to 8 minutes longer or until golden brown and heated through. Serve immediately.

Alternatively, spray a nonstick skillet with olive oil spray and set the pan over medium-high heat for about 2 minutes to heat. Put the patties in the pan and cook for 2 to 3 minutes on each side or until golden brown and heated through.

NUTRITIONAL ANALYSIS (per serving):
Total carbohydrates: 27 g / Protein: 10 g / Fat: 8 g / Dietary fiber: 7 g / Calories: 210

The Pump Restaurant makes eating healthy a no-brainer. My favorite meal after a great workout is #43, the Pizza-Style Turkey Burger, with a mixed vegetable juice and sweet potato pie. I also enjoy the omelets, pancakes, Baseball, and falafel sandwich. I keep my workouts strong but simple. I try anything new to see how it affects my body ... but always go back to the basics. A strong foundation is your best ally for life. I also believe gratitude is the best motivation. I'm grateful to be alive and healthy.

—MARIA DiGIUSEPPE, Elegante Fitness

Rookie Steak Burger

EVERYONE LOVES BURGERS AND THIS ONE SCORES BIG POINTS with our customers. The simple tomato and cucumber topping make this burger a bold and full-flavored meal—you'll never miss the fries! When you buy ground beef, look for ground sirloin, which is far leaner than ground chuck, the meat most commonly marketed for hamburgers. We serve the burger in pita bread, but you'll still need a fork.

SERVES 1

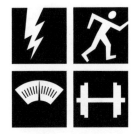

¼ cup **THE PUMP'S HOMEMADE TOMATO SAUCE**, page 110

¼ cup minced **CUCUMBER**

3 tablespoons minced **TOMATO**

2 tablespoons minced **ONION**

1 teaspoon dried **OREGANO**

6 ounces lean **GROUND SIRLOIN**

3 ounces nonfat **MOZZARELLA**, shredded (about 1 cup)

1 whole wheat 5-inch **PITA BREAD**, toasted

In a small bowl, combine the tomato sauce, cucumber, tomato, onion, and oregano and stir to mix. You will have about ¾ cup of the mixture.

Form the ground meat into a patty about 1 inch thick. Set a medium nonstick skillet over medium-high heat and cook the burger for 4 minutes. Turn and cook for 2 to 3 minutes longer for medium rare. Pour the vegetables over and around the burger and sprinkle with the cheese. Cover the pan and cook for 3 to 5 minutes or until the vegetables are heated through and the cheese melts.

Serve the burger in the pita bread, with the vegetables spooned over it.

NUTRITIONAL ANALYSIS (per serving):
Total carbohydrates: 35 g / Protein: 65 g / Fat: 9 g / Dietary fiber: 7 g / Calories: 490

When you think of eating healthfully, the first thoughts that come to mind are bland and boring. Well, not at the Pump. I've been eating lunch there for the past six months and I love it! I can't even think of eating fast food again. I no longer feel fatigued in the afternoon; I feel full of energy.
—JAMES FILATRO

Pizza-Style Turkey Burger

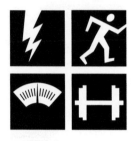

PUMP REGULARS LOVE THIS BURGER. They tell us that when they get a hankering for a fast food burger, they buy one of these instead. And they are always glad when they do. It's a perfect alternative to fast food.

SERVES 1

6 ounces **GROUND TURKEY BREAST**

1 whole wheat 5-inch **PITA BREAD**, toasted and split in half

3 tablespoons **THE PUMP'S HOMEMADE TOMATO SAUCE**, page 110

3 ounces nonfat **MOZZARELLA**, shredded (about 1 cup)

Pinch dried **OREGANO**

Preheat the oven to 425°F.

Form the ground turkey into a patty about 1 inch thick. Set a nonstick skillet over medium-high heat and cook the burger for 4 minutes. Turn and cook for 3 to 5 minutes longer or until the juices run clear.

Put the burger on the pita. Spread 2 tablespoons of tomato sauce on the burger and then top with the cheese. Spoon the final tablespoon of sauce over the cheese and sprinkle with oregano. Press the pita closed, transfer to a baking pan, and bake for 5 to 6 minutes or until the cheese melts. Serve immediately.

NUTRITIONAL ANALYSIS (per serving):
Total carbohydrates: 34 g / Protein: 73 g / Fat: 5 g / Dietary fiber: 6 g / Calories: 480

PUMP LIFESTYLE REASONS PEOPLE ARE OVERWEIGHT

Fattening food is cheap.

Fattening food is everywhere.

Fattening food is designed to be eaten easily and in big quantities.

You barely have to even chew it.

Food served at most events is often full of empty carbohydrates.

Food served at most school cafeterias is highly processed and full of saturated fat.

Food is often manipulated so that it can look better and last forever without regard for its nutritional value.

09.
Vegetable Sides

Steamed Green and White Vegetables / Roasted Cinnamon Squash / Dill-and-Chive Snow Peas and Carrots / Baked Zucchini / Warm Asparagus and Snow Pea Salad / Tomato Stacks / Sautéed Sugar Snap Peas with Mushrooms / Quinoa with Dill / Crispy Sliced Potatoes / Eggplant Carpaccio / Spinach with Feta Cheese / Simply Cooked Sweet Potatoes / Brown Rice with Peas and Carrots / Sautéed Sliced Mushrooms with Sun-dried Tomatoes

Steamed Green and White Vegetables

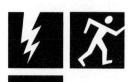

HOW OFTEN HAVE YOU SEEN AN ADVERTISEMENT FOR BROCCOLI OR CAULIFLOWER? Not too often! But once you start working this side dish into your weekly diet, you will become a walking commercial for the goodness of these steamed vegetables. Eating this alongside fish, chicken, or steak leaves you feeling cleansed and satisfied, yet never stuffed.

SERVES 4

1/2 bunch **BROCCOLI**, cut into florets, thick stems discarded (about 3/4 pound of broccoli)

1/2 head **CAULIFLOWER**, cut into florets (about 3/4 pound of cauliflower)

2 small **ZUCCHINI**, trimmed and sliced (about 3/4 pound)

1 small **CARROT**, trimmed, peeled, and sliced

ZEST OF 1 LEMON, finely grated

Chop the broccoli and cauliflower florets into bite-size pieces.

In a steamer basket set over boiling water or in an electric steamer, steam the vegetables for 3 to 5 minutes, or until fork-tender. Serve the steamed vegetables sprinkled with zest.

VARIATION: Substitute 1 cup of thinly sliced snow peas for the carrots. You could also substitute 3/4 pound of trimmed and halved wax beans or string beans for the carrots.

NUTRITIONAL ANALYSIS (per serving):
Total carbohydrates: 10 g / Protein: 4 g / Fat: .5 g / Dietary fiber: 5 g / Calories: 50

Roasted Cinnamon Squash

THIS DISH IS ONE OF OUR FAVORITES TO COOK IN THE FALL when we first see butternut squash in the markets. It takes time but is warm, nourishing, and so sweet, you could almost eat it for dessert! The toasted pumpkin seeds make a great snack on their own.

SERVES 6

OLIVE OIL COOKING SPRAY

3¼ pounds **BUTTERNUT SQUASH**

2 tablespoons ground **CINNAMON**

½ cup raw shelled **PUMPKIN SEEDS** (pepitas)

¼ teaspoon **SEA SALT**, optional

⅛ teaspoon **CAYENNE**

⅛ teaspoon **ALLSPICE**

Preheat the oven to 400°F. Spray a large, shallow baking pan with olive oil cooking spray.

Cut the squash in half and scoop out the soft interior and seeds.

Lay the squash pieces skin side up in the baking pan and roast for 20 to 25 minutes or until the flesh is softened enough to make it easy to peel the flesh from the shell.

Let the squash cool for 10 or 15 minutes, or until cool enough to handle. Peel off and discard the outer shell. Slice the squash into large chunks and arrange them in a single layer on the baking pan. Sprinkle with cinnamon. Roast for about 20 to 25 minutes or until the squash is very soft and glazed with the cinnamon.

Meanwhile, toast the seeds in a dry, nonstick skillet over medium heat for 2 to 3 minutes, shaking the pan, until lightly golden and puffed. Add the salt, if using, cayenne, and allspice and stir to mix.

Serve the squash sprinkled with the seeds.

NUTRITIONAL ANALYSIS (per serving):

Total carbohydrates: 31 g / Protein: 5 g / Fat: 6 g / Dietary fiber: 5 g / Calories: 170

Dill-and-Chive Snow Peas and Carrots

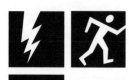

SNOW PEAS ARE CRUNCHY AND GOOD, and never more so than when mixed with carrots. We flavor this with dill and it's great with fish or chicken.

SERVES 6

4 cups **WATER**

2 medium **CARROTS**, peeled and cut into 2-inch-long matchsticks (about 2 cups)

4 to 5 cups trimmed **SNOW PEAS** (about 1 pound)

3 tablespoons minced **CHIVES**

3 teaspoons minced fresh **DILL**

In a large saucepan, bring the water to a boil over high heat. Add the carrots, reduce the heat to a rapid simmer, and cook for 2 minutes or until the carrots begin to soften. Add the snow peas and cook for 1 to 2 minutes longer or until both vegetables are crisp-tender.

Drain through a colander and return the vegetables to the hot pan. Add the chives and dill, toss gently, and serve.

NUTRITIONAL ANALYSIS (per serving):
Total carbohydrates: 7 g / Protein: 2 g / Fat: 0 g / Dietary fiber: 2 g / Calories: 40

Baked Zucchini

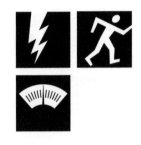

IF YOU LIKE DEEP-FRIED ZUCCHINI, YOU WILL LOVE THIS DISH! It's much better than deep-fried squash, which soaks up oil; in this recipe you get all the flavor and texture without the oil. Keep your eye on the zucchini while it bakes, as it burns easily.

SERVES 4

4 medium **ZUCCHINI**, ends trimmed, cut into
    ¼-inch-thick rounds

OLIVE OIL COOKING SPRAY

3 tablespoons **DRIED ONION-PARSLEY MIX**,
    such as Mrs. Dash

1 medium **CARROT**, peeled, trimmed, and
    coarsely shredded

Preheat the oven to 350°F.

Put the zucchini in a large mixing bowl and spray lightly with olive oil spray. Toss to coat. Sprinkle with the onion-parsley mix and toss again.

Spread the zucchini rounds in a large, shallow nonstick baking pan. Bake on the bottom shelf of the oven for 20 to 30 minutes, or until golden. Stir the vegetables 2 or 3 times as they bake.

Remove the pan from the oven and sprinkle the shredded carrot over the zucchini. Return the pan to the oven and bake for 5 to 10 minutes longer or until the carrots start to brown and soften. Serve immediately.

NUTRITIONAL ANALYSIS (per serving):
Total carbohydrates: 8 g / Protein: 3 g / Fat: 1 g / Dietary fiber: 3 g / Calories: 40

Warm Asparagus and Snow Pea Salad

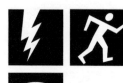

SERVE THIS SALAD WITH A SIMPLE PROTEIN such as grilled chicken or broiled fish. We eat asparagus four or five times per week, partly because it's so good for you but mostly for its taste. Snow peas are also delicious and refreshing. When you clean asparagus, bend the stalks gently; they will break naturally where they need to be trimmed.

SERVES 4

8 medium stalks **ASPARAGUS**

1 cup thinly sliced **CARROTS** (sliced on the diagonal)

4 slender ribs **CELERY**, sliced

2½ ounces **SNOW PEAS**, cleaned and trimmed

4 tablespoons **DRY WHITE WINE**

2 tablespoons extra-virgin **OLIVE OIL**

2 tablespoons **WHITE WINE VINEGAR**

1 tablespoon chopped fresh **DILL**

Pinch of **SEA SALT**, optional

Freshly ground **BLACK PEPPER**, optional

Break the tough ends from the asparagus stalks (they should break where they naturally bend). Discard the ends. Peel the stalks and cut each into lengths about 3 inches long.

In an electric steamer or a steamer basket set over boiling water, steam the carrots and celery for about 4 minutes or until they begin to soften. Add the asparagus and snow peas and continue steaming for 3 to 4 minutes longer or until all the vegetables are fork-tender. Drain and transfer to a bowl.

Meanwhile, whisk together the wine, olive oil, vinegar, and dill. Season to taste with salt and pepper, if desired.

Pour the dressing over the hot vegetables, toss gently, and let sit for about 30 minutes before serving warm.

NUTRITIONAL ANALYSIS (per serving):
Total carbohydrates: 7 g / Protein: 2 g / Fat: 7 g / Dietary fiber: 2 g / Calories: 110

Tomato Stacks

LIGHTLY BROILED, CHEESE-KISSED "TOMATO SANDWICHES" ARE A TREAT. We love them in the summer when the tomatoes are at their very best. Add a few thin slices of cooked chicken to the stacks for a light main course, or serve these as a side dish with any plainly cooked chicken, beef, lamb, or fish.

SERVES 4

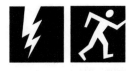

OLIVE OIL COOKING SPRAY

2 large ripe **TOMATOES**

1¼ cups shredded nonfat **MOZZARELLA** (about 4 ounces)

1 tablespoon grated high-quality **PARMESAN CHEESE**

8 or 9 **KALAMATA OLIVES**, pitted and sliced

12 fresh **BASIL LEAVES**, washed, dried, and roughly torn

2 teaspoons **BALSAMIC VINEGAR**

Preheat the broiler. Spray the broiling pan with olive oil cooking spray.

Core the tomatoes and slice each crosswise into 4 even slices. Lay 4 of the tomato slices on the broiling pan and sprinkle with half the mozzarella and all the Parmesan cheese. Sprinkle with olives and basil leaves and top with the remaining tomato slices.

Broil about 6 inches from the heat for about 5 minutes or until the cheese melts.

Remove the broiling pan and sprinkle the top tomato slices with the rest of the cheese. Broil for about 2 minutes longer or until the cheese melts over the top of the tomato stacks. Using a spatula, transfer the tomato stacks to a serving platter and drizzle each with about ½ teaspoon of vinegar.

NUTRITIONAL ANALYSIS (per serving):
Total carbohydrates: 4 g / Protein: 10 g / Fat: 3 g / Dietary fiber: 1 g / Calories: 80

Sautéed Sugar Snap Peas with Mushrooms

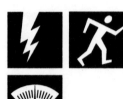

THIS QUICK STIR-FRY INCLUDES MANY OF OUR FAVORITE VEGETABLES—sugar snap peas, mushrooms, leeks, and bell peppers—flavored with ginger, garlic, and some Braggs Liquid Aminos for an Asian flair. The amino acids are available in health food stores and many other markets, but if you can't locate them, substitute a low-sodium soy sauce. Don't be alarmed by the number of ingredients; they all complement each other and result in a light, refreshing side dish.

SERVES 4

2 tablespoons **BRAGGS LIQUID AMINOS** or low-sodium **SOY SAUCE**

2 tablespoons **WHITE BALSAMIC VINEGAR**

One 1-inch piece fresh **GINGER**, peeled and grated

2 small cloves **GARLIC**, minced

1 medium **LEEK**, white part only, sliced

1/2 pound **WHITE** or **CREMINI MUSHROOMS**, sliced (about 3 cups)

1/2 cup chopped **YELLOW BELL PEPPER**

1 pound **SUGAR SNAP PEAS**, trimmed (about 4 cups)

2 to 3 tablespoons **WATER**

1 to 2 **SCALLIONS**, white and pale green parts, minced, optional

In a wok set over medium-high heat, combine the amino acids and vinegar. Add the ginger and garlic and stir-fry for about 30 seconds or until fragrant.

Add the leek, mushrooms, and pepper, reduce the heat to medium low, and stir-fry for 2 to 3 minutes or until the mushrooms begin to release their liquid. Add the sugar snap peas, mix well, and stir-fry for 8 to 10 minutes or until the vegetables are tender. Add the water during final minutes of cooking for moisture. Serve right away garnished with scallions, if desired.

NUTRITIONAL ANALYSIS (per serving):
Total carbohydrates: 18 g / Protein: 5 g / Fat: .5 g / Dietary fiber: 4 g / Calories: 90

Quinoa with Dill

AS WE HAVE SAID IN OTHER RECIPES WITH QUINOA (page 100), we love this complex carbo-hydrate. It cooks more quickly than brown rice and is just as nutritious, earning its reputation as a good carb. When you add dill, the quinoa perks up and turns into a versatile side dish.
SERVES 4

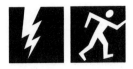

2 cups **WATER**

1 cup **QUINOA**

3 tablespoons chopped fresh **DILL**
(about 15 sprigs)

In a saucepan, bring the water to a boil over high heat. Stir in the quinoa, reduce the heat to medium low, and cook, partially covered, for about 15 minutes or until the water is absorbed.

Remove the quinoa from the heat and stir in the dill. Serve right away.

NUTRITIONAL ANALYSIS (per serving):
Total carbohydrates: 29 g / Protein: 6 g / Fat: 2.5 g / Dietary fiber: 3 g / Calories: 160

Crispy Sliced Potatoes

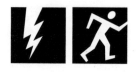

IF YOU OFTEN HUNGER FOR FRENCH FRIES, these will satisfy those cravings. Once you start eating our version, greasy fries will taste of nothing but grease and salt! With these, you can really taste the potatoes. Eat them as a snack or a side dish. Make some extras and reheat them in the microwave.

SERVES 4

4 medium **BAKING POTATOES**
OLIVE OIL COOKING SPRAY

SEA SALT, optional

Soak the potatoes in warm water for 15 minutes. Remove and scrub with a vegetable brush to remove all dirt. Rinse under cool, running water.

Bring a large saucepan filled about two-thirds full with water to a boil over high heat. Add the potatoes, reduce the heat to medium high, and simmer for 30 minutes or until the potatoes begin to soften. Do not cook until tender. Drain for about 15 minutes to give them time to dry out a little.

Preheat the oven to 400°F.

Cut each potato lengthwise into 5 or 6 thick slices and spread in a single layer on a nonstick baking pan or sheet. Spray lightly with cooking spray.

Bake for about 15 minutes, turning once or twice, until crispy on the outside. Serve sprinkled with a little salt, if desired.

NUTRITIONAL ANALYSIS (per serving):
Total carbohydrates: 26 g / Protein: 4 g / Fat: .5 g / Dietary fiber: 3 g / Calories: 100

Eggplant Carpaccio

AS A BASE FOR ALL SORTS OF GOOD TOPPINGS, NOTHING BEATS EGGPLANT. It is firm enough, has fantastic flavor, and is easy to work with. We admit this is not really a classic carpaccio, a dish consisting of thinly sliced raw meat or fish served with a sauce. Instead it's a delicious side dish made with thinly sliced, lightly cooked eggplant topped with some of the garden's tastiest bounty and a little cheese. As good as it is as a side dish, it also makes a lovely appetizer.

SERVES 4

OLIVE OIL COOKING SPRAY

1 medium **EGGPLANT** (about 1½ pounds), peeled and sliced crosswise in ¼- to ½-inch-thick slices

2 **PLUM TOMATOES**, chopped

¼ cup diced **RED ONION**

¼ cup packed minced **FLAT-LEAF PARSLEY** (about ¼ bunch)

1 teaspoon **BALSAMIC VINEGAR**

1 teaspoon **OLIVE OIL**

1 small clove **GARLIC**, minced

2½ ounces shredded low-fat **MOZZARELLA** (about ¾ cup)

Preheat the oven to 450°F. Spray a 10-by-15-inch jelly roll pan with cooking spray.

Lay the eggplant slices in a single layer in the pan and spray lightly with cooking spray. Bake for 15 minutes or until softened and golden on the bottom. Turn slices and cook for about 15 minutes longer or until golden on both sides.

Meanwhile, in a small bowl, stir together the tomatoes, onion, and parsley. Add the vinegar, olive oil, and garlic and stir gently.

Remove the cooked eggplant from the oven, turn slices over, and move them closer together. Sprinkle with ½ cup of the shredded cheese. Spoon the tomato mixture over the cheese and then top with the remaining ¼ cup cheese. Bake for about 5 minutes longer, or until the cheese melts and the tomatoes are heated through. Serve right from the oven or let the eggplant cool slightly.

The Pump has delicious food that keeps me going throughout the day. I never feel tired or hyper after eating there because the food seems to have the proper balance of carbohydrates, protein, and other essential nutrients. The menu suits many different tastes from hard-core meat eaters to vegetarians and vegans and keeps expanding with a variety of delicious things to eat.

—JENIERE D. BAILEY

NUTRITIONAL ANALYSIS (per serving):

Total carbohydrates: 16 g / Protein: 4 g / Fat: 3.5 g / Dietary fiber: 1 g / Calories: 100

Spinach with Feta Cheese

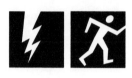

THIS DISH IS REMINISCENT OF THE FLAVORS FOUND IN A TRADITIONAL Greek spinach pie. We prefer the flavor of fresh spinach. Nowadays the spinach sold in bags is not as sandy as fresh spinach used to be, so it is easier to clean. Drain the spinach if it seems watery after steaming.

SERVES 6

OLIVE OIL COOKING SPRAY
Two 10-ounce bags **SPINACH LEAVES**, washed
1 large **YELLOW ONION**, diced

$1/3$ cup chopped fresh **DILL** (about $1/4$ bunch)
4 ounces low-fat **FETA**, crumbled
2 teaspoons dried **OREGANO**

Preheat the oven to 475°F. Spray a shallow 9-by-13-inch baking pan with cooking spray.

In a steamer basket over boiling water or in an electric steamer, steam the spinach for 3 to 5 minutes or until wilted. Drain if necessary.

Spread the onion in the baking pan and bake for 10 to 15 minutes or until somewhat softened, lightly brown, and fragrant. Stir the onions several times during cooking.

Spread the wilted spinach over the onions and then sprinkle the dill over the spinach. Scatter the feta over the top and sprinkle with oregano. Return the pan to the oven and bake for 8 to 10 minutes or until the cheese browns lightly and the vegetables are hot.

NUTRITIONAL ANALYSIS (per serving):
Total carbohydrates: 7 g / Protein: 7 g / Fat: 2.5 g / Dietary fiber: 2 g / Calories: 70

Simply Cooked Sweet Potatoes

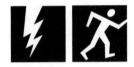

WHEN YOU WORK OUT, YOU NEED GOOD COMPLEX CARBOHYDRATES, such as sweet potatoes and brown rice. They give you energy. We like these warm or cold, even for breakfast or as a snack. They are excellent accompaniments to proteins such as chicken and tuna, too. We cook several and keep them in the refrigerator for two or three days. Store them in a colander set on a plate to keep them dry with air circulating around them.

SERVES 4

4 medium **SWEET POTATOES** or **YAMS**
(about 1/2 pound)

Soak the potatoes in warm water for 15 minutes. Remove and scrub with a vegetable brush to remove all dirt. Rinse under cool, running water.

Bring a large saucepan filled about two-thirds full with water to a boil over high heat. Add the potatoes, reduce the heat to medium low, and simmer, partially covered, for 50 to 60 minutes or until the potatoes are tender when pricked with the tip of a small sharp knife. Drain for about 15 minutes so all the water drains.

Eat while still warm. To store, refrigerate for up to 3 days. Store them in a colander to allow air to circulate.

NUTRITIONAL ANALYSIS (per serving):
Total carbohydrates: 24 g / Protein: 2 g / Fat: 0 g / Dietary fiber: 4 g / Calories: 100

Brown Rice with Peas and Carrots

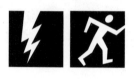

BROWN RICE IS GREAT, but it's advisable to eat complex carbohydrates like it and sweet potatoes during the day—for breakfast, lunch, or as a snack. They really keep you going. You don't need the energy they provide in the evening before bed. Brown rice is endlessly versatile and when mixed with vegetables just gets better. The dill really peps this dish up.

SERVES 4

⅓ cup plus 2 tablespoons **WATER**

1 **YELLOW ONION**, diced

2 medium **CARROTS**, trimmed, peeled, and coarsely shredded

½ cup fresh or frozen **GREEN PEAS**

1 tablespoon chopped fresh **DILL**

2 cups hot cooked **BROWN RICE**, page 139

SEA SALT, optional

In a saucepan, cook the onion and 2 tablespoons of water over medium-low heat, covered and stirring occasionally to prevent sticking, for 4 to 5 minutes until slightly softened. Add the carrots and cook, covered and stirring occasionally, for about 2 minutes until carrots start to soften.

Add the remaining ⅓ cup of water and peas and cook over medium heat, uncovered, for 3 to 5 minutes or until the vegetables are tender and the liquid has reduced to about 2 tablespoons.

Stir the vegetables and dill into the rice, season with salt if using, and serve.

NUTRITIONAL ANALYSIS (per serving):
Total carbohydrates: 32 g / Protein: 4 g / Fat: 1 g / Dietary fiber: 5 g / Calories: 150

Sautéed Sliced Mushrooms with Sun-dried Tomatoes

WE LOVE THE FLAVOR OF MUSHROOMS, which only improves with cooking. Paired with sun-dried tomatoes, garlic, and capers, mushrooms become an elegant side dish that does justice to grilled, broiled, or oven-baked chicken or beef.

SERVES 4

¹/₄ cup **WHITE WINE VINEGAR**
2 tablespoons low-sodium **SOY SAUCE**
2 cloves **GARLIC**, chopped
2 tablespoons drained **CAPERS**
5 oil-packed **SUN-DRIED TOMATOES**, chopped

3 cups sliced **WHITE** or **CREMINI MUSHROOMS** (about 10 ounces)
1 tablespoon **DRIED ONION-PARSLEY MIX**, such as Mrs. Dash

In a large nonstick skillet or wok, heat the vinegar and soy sauce over medium-high heat. Add the garlic, capers, and sun-dried tomatoes and stir-fry for about 1 minute. Add the mushrooms and stir-fry for 2 to 3 minutes or until the mushrooms begin to soften.

Cover the wok, reduce the heat to low, and cook for 3 minutes. Season with onion-parsley mixture, stir, cover, and cook for 2 to 4 minutes longer, or until the mushrooms are soft and flavorful and most of the excess liquid evaporates. Serve immediately.

NUTRITIONAL ANALYSIS (per serving):
Total carbohydrates: 6 g / Protein: 2 g / Fat: .5 g / Dietary fiber: 1 g / Calories: 35

STEAMING SPINACH

Wash two 10-ounce bags of baby spinach or spinach leaves well.

Shake dry, leaving some water clinging to the leaves.

Steam in a steamer basket set over boiling water or in an electric steamer for 3 to 5 minutes.

Drain if necessary.

Makes approximately 2 cups steamed spinach.

COOKING BROWN RICE

Pour 1 cup of brown rice into a saucepan containing $2^1/_2$ cups of boiling water. Stir once, cover the pan, and reduce the heat to low.

Cook for 35 to 45 minutes, or until all the water is absorbed.

Let the rice stand, still covered, for about 5 minutes.

Fluff with a fork and serve. You will have about $3^1/_2$ cups of cooked rice.

10.
Pump Shakes and Juices

Strawberry-Banana Shake / Frozen Banana Shake / Carrot-Orange Shake / Strawberry Shake / Creamy Orange-Banana Meal-Substitute Shake / Apple-Strawberry Shake / Summer Shake / Thick Coffee Shake / Peaches-and-Cream Shake / Papaya Protein Shake / Banana–Peanut Butter Chocolate Shake / Tropical Island Shake / Summer Berry Shake / Mixed Fruit Shake / Chocolate Whey Protein Shake / The Pump Energy Shake / Banana-Strawberry Soy Protein Shake / Blueberry-Apple Protein Shake / Creativity Juice / Get-Up-and-Go Juice / Carrot-Apple-Celery Juice / Grapefruit-Orange Juice

WE MAKE ALL OF OUR SHAKES FOR THE SAME REASON: They taste great and make you feel terrific. They are perfect as between-meal snacks, meal substitutes, and alternatives to dessert. We're also known for our delicious freshly squeezed juices, great for a healthful burst of energy. Each of the four we offer at the end of this chapter has been popular at the Pump since we opened.

When you make the fruit shakes, be sure the fruit is ripe or even a little overripe. We like to chill fresh fruit before we blend it, but this step is not crucial. High-quality frozen fruit is a good choice, too, particularly if the fresh fruit in your markets is not good (a problem in the wintertime). Read the labels before buying frozen fruit and berries to make sure they are not packaged with sugar or syrup. The shake's sweetness depends on the sweetness of the fruit.

Shakes fortified with protein provide an awesome energy boost! After even a few sips, you start to feel great. If you are unfamiliar with protein powders, using them in shakes is a good way to try them. All brands share a lot of similarities, but they also differ slightly one from another, too. Try several different brands until you find the one you like. They come in different flavors, and for our shakes, we generally use vanilla protein powder.

If you are unsure about them, start with less powder than our recipe or the package recommends. Add more as you go along. Steve likes a powder called Designer Protein powder, which is whey-based (for a treat, he sprinkles chocolate Designer Protein powder over plain yogurt), and we both like Spirutein, which is soy-based (we sprinkle this over our morning oatmeal). You'll have to find the brand you like.

If you haven't tried protein powders in several years, take heart. They are much improved and really taste good.

We suggest drinking our shakes as between-meal lifts and treats, although the protein shakes can serve as meal replacements. None of these is meant to accompany a meal—drink water with meals—but could be served as dessert.

Most of our recipes are for a single serving, but since they yield about two cups, you could easily turn these into two smaller servings. We use standard-size ice cubes, which measure about 1/2 cup of water for every 6 cubes. Break up the ice cubes before adding them to the blender for smoother, easier processing and remove any ice chunks that float after blending.

To make our shakes, you will need a blender. The better the blender, the smoother the shakes and the more likely you will be to make shakes with regularity, so invest in a good one. You don't have to buy the best on the market, but don't go hunting in bargain basements!

For the juices, you need a juice extractor. These machines are pricier than blenders, but since their purpose is to remove the juice from the vegetables or fruit and leave nothing behind for disposal but nearly dry pulp, they must be powerful. You cannot use a blender to make juice. When you use a juice extractor, there is no need to stem, peel, seed, or core the fruit (citrus fruit is the exception; these do better when peeled to keep the juice from tasting bitter). Wash the vegetables and fruit well and then cut them up only as needed to fit through the feeder tube. The juice is best if drunk as soon as it's extracted.

Strawberry-Banana Shake

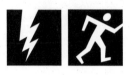

SERVES 1; MAKES ABOUT 2 CUPS

¹/₂ ripe **BANANA**, sliced (about ¹/₂ cup)

5 fresh or frozen **STRAWBERRIES,** rinsed and trimmed if fresh, quartered

8 **ICE CUBES**, roughly broken

¹/₂ cup **NONFAT FROZEN YOGURT** or **SORBET** (1 generous scoop)

³/₄ cup **APPLE JUICE**

Put the banana, strawberries, ice cubes, yogurt, and apple juice in the canister of a blender. Blend until smooth. Serve immediately.

NUTRITIONAL ANALYSIS (per serving):

Total carbohydrates: 54 g / Protein: 7 g / Fat: .5 g / Dietary fiber: 3 g / Calories: 240

Frozen Banana Shake

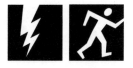

SERVES 1; MAKES ABOUT 2 CUPS

1 large frozen **BANANA**, see Note
²/₃ cup **SKIM MILK**
6 **ICE CUBES**, roughly broken

¹/₂ cup nonfat **VANILLA FROZEN YOGURT**
(1 generous scoop)

Put the frozen banana, skim milk, ice cubes, and yogurt in the canister of a blender. Blend until smooth. Serve immediately.

NOTE: To freeze the banana, peel it and wrap in plastic wrap or enclose in a plastic bag. Freeze for at least 3 hours and up to 24 hours, or until frozen solid.

NUTRITIONAL ANALYSIS (per serving):
Total carbohydrates: 55 g / Protein: 12 g / Fat: .5 g / Dietary fiber: 3 g / Calories: 260

Carrot-Orange Shake

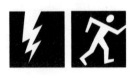

SERVES 1; MAKES ABOUT 2 CUPS

8 **ICE CUBES**, roughly broken

1/2 cup **ORANGE JUICE**

1/3 cup **CARROT JUICE**, see Note

1/2 cup nonfat **VANILLA FROZEN YOGURT** (1 generous scoop)

Put the ice cubes, orange juice, carrot juice, and yogurt in the canister of a blender. Blend until smooth. Serve immediately.

NOTE: You can buy carrot juice from a health food store or juice bar or make your own if you have a juice extractor. Store-bought or homemade, carrot juice does not store well, so buy or make it on the same day you want to make the shake.

NUTRITIONAL ANALYSIS (per serving):
Total carbohydrates: 36 g / Protein: 6 g / Fat: .5 g / Dietary fiber: 0 g / Calories: 170

Strawberry Shake

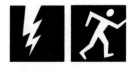

SERVES 1; MAKES ABOUT 2 CUPS

8 large fresh or frozen **STRAWBERRIES**, rinsed and trimmed if fresh, quartered

1/2 cup **SKIM MILK**

8 **ICE CUBES**, roughly broken

1/2 cup nonfat **VANILLA FROZEN YOGURT** (1 generous scoop)

Put the strawberries, skim milk, ice cubes, and yogurt in the canister of a blender. Blend until smooth. Serve immediately.

NUTRITIONAL ANALYSIS (per serving):
Total carbohydrates: 37 g / Protein: 10 g / Fat: .5 g / Dietary fiber: 3 g / Calories: 190

Creamy Orange-Banana Meal-Substitute Shake

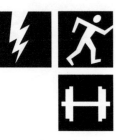

I work a 90+ hour work week, and somehow I manage to fit in an hour workout every day. The only thing that keeps me energized throughout my workout is the Pump's food! My body reacts very strongly to salt, oils, and fatty foods. The Pump has found a way to replace the salt and fat with flavor, so now I feel lighter on my feet. I'm not as hungry as before, and I have so much more energy when I work out. Thank you, Pump!
—WILEY B. CERILLI

SERVES 1; MAKES ABOUT 2 CUPS

½ large frozen **BANANA**

⅔ cup of **ORANGE JUICE**

⅓ cup of **SKIM MILK** or **RICE MILK**

6 **ICE CUBES**, roughly broken

1 package (2.7 ounces) of **PROTEIN AND CARBOHYDRATE POWDER**

Put the frozen banana, orange juice, milk, and ice cubes in the canister of a blender. Blend for a few seconds. Add the protein powder and blend until smooth. Use a rubber spatula to push the protein powder into the shake. Serve immediately.

NOTE: To freeze the banana, peel it and wrap in plastic wrap or enclose in a plastic bag. Freeze for at least 3 hours and up to 24 hours, or until frozen solid.

NUTRITIONAL ANALYSIS (per serving):

Total carbohydrates: 58 g / Protein: 47 g / Fat: 3 g / Dietary fiber: 5 g / Calories: 420

Apple-Strawberry Shake

SERVES 1; MAKES ABOUT 2 CUPS

10 large fresh or frozen **STRAWBERRIES**, rinsed and trimmed if fresh, quartered

10 **ICE CUBES**, roughly broken

1/2 cup **APPLE JUICE**

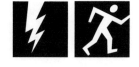

Put the strawberries, ice cubes, and apple juice in the canister of a blender. Blend until smooth. Serve immediately.

NUTRITIONAL ANALYSIS (per serving):
Total carbohydrates: 28 g / Protein: 2 g / Fat: .5 g / Dietary fiber: 4 g / Calories: 120

Summer Shake

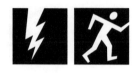

SERVES 1; MAKES ABOUT 2 CUPS

8 large fresh or frozen **STRAWBERRIES**, rinsed
and trimmed if fresh, quartered

8 **ICE CUBES**, roughly broken

1/2 cup homemade or frozen and reconstituted
LEMONADE, see Note

1/2 cup nonfat **VANILLA FROZEN YOGURT** or
LEMON or **ORANGE SORBET** (1 generous
scoop)

Put the strawberries, ice cubes, lemonade, and yogurt in the canister of a blender. Blend until smooth. Serve immediately.

NOTE: You can substitute reconstituted powdered lemonade, such as Crystal Light, for the fresh or frozen lemonade.

NUTRITIONAL ANALYSIS (per serving):
Total carbohydrates: 37 g / Protein: 6 g / Fat: .5 g / Dietary fiber: 3 g / Calories: 170

Thick Coffee Shake

SERVES 1; MAKES ABOUT 2 CUPS

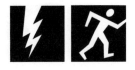

²/₃ cup **SKIM MILK, RICE MILK,** or **SOY MILK**

2 teaspoons instant **COFFEE** or **ESPRESSO GRANULES**

1 teaspoon **SUGAR** or **SPLENDA** or another granulated **SUGAR SUBSTITUTE**

8 **ICE CUBES**, roughly broken

½ cup nonfat **COFFEE FROZEN YOGURT** (1 generous scoop)

Put the milk, coffee granules, sugar, ice cubes, and frozen yogurt in the canister of a blender. Blend until smooth. Serve immediately.

NUTRITIONAL ANALYSIS (per serving):

Total carbohydrates: 30 g / Protein: 11 g / Fat: 0 g / Dietary fiber: 0 g / Calories: 170

Peaches-and-Cream Shake

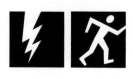

1 cup cubed fresh or frozen **PEACHES**,
see Note
4 **ICE CUBES**, roughly broken
1/2 cup **ORANGE JUICE**

1/3 cup **SKIM MILK**
1/2 cup nonfat **VANILLA FROZEN YOGURT**
(1 generous scoop)

Put the peaches, ice cubes, orange juice, milk, and yogurt in the canister of a blender. Blend until smooth. Serve immediately.

NOTE: Look for frozen IQF fruit, which is very high quality and does not contain syrup or added sugar. It's easy to find in supermarkets.

NUTRITIONAL ANALYSIS (per serving):
Total carbohydrates: 52 g / Protein: 10 g / Fat: .5 g / Dietary fiber: 0 g / Calories: 250

Papaya Protein Shake

SERVES 1; MAKES ABOUT 2 CUPS

4 ounces **PAPAYA**, cut into cubes

10 **ICE CUBES**, roughly broken

²/₃ cup **ORANGE JUICE**

1 scoop **VANILLA PROTEIN POWDER**
(about ¹/₄ cup), see Note

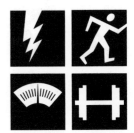

Put the papaya, ice cubes, and orange juice in the canister of a blender. With the motor running, add the protein powder. Blend until thick and smooth. Serve immediately.

NOTE: Protein powder makes shakes thick. You may have to stir the shake with a rubber spatula when partly blended and then continue blending.

NUTRITIONAL ANALYSIS (per serving):
Total carbohydrates: 30 g / Protein: 18.5 g / Fat: 1.5 g / Dietary fiber: 2.5 g / Calories: 210

One day . . . I tried the Pump after a workout and loved it. After that, I made trips to the Pump part of my workout routine, whether [I ordered] a smoothie or a Supercharged Plate. The Pump helped me to reach my goal and, more important, maintain my weight.

—MANUEL VEGA

Banana-Peanut Butter Chocolate Shake

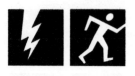

SERVES 1; MAKES ABOUT 2 CUPS

1 large ripe **BANANA**

1 tablespoon natural **CREAMY PEANUT BUTTER**

8 **ICE CUBES**, roughly broken

1/2 cup **SKIM MILK, RICE MILK,** or **SOY MILK**

1/2 cup nonfat **CHOCOLATE FROZEN YOGURT** (1 generous scoop)

Put the banana, peanut butter, ice cubes, milk, and yogurt in the canister of a blender. Blend until smooth. Serve immediately.

NUTRITIONAL ANALYSIS (per serving):

Total carbohydrates: 56 g / Protein: 14 g / Fat: 9 g / Dietary fiber: 4 g / Calories: 350

Tropical Island Shake

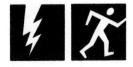

5 ounces **CANTALOUPE**, cut into small chunks (about 1½ cups)

½ ripe **MANGO**, diced

8 **ICE CUBES**, roughly broken

¼ cup **APPLE JUICE**

⅓ cup **SKIM MILK**, **RICE MILK**, or **SOY MILK**

Put the cantaloupe, mango, ice cubes, apple juice, and milk in the canister of a blender. Blend until smooth. Serve immediately.

NUTRITIONAL ANALYSIS (per serving):
Total carbohydrates: 40 g / Protein: 4 g / Fat: 1 g / Dietary fiber: 1 g / Calories: 180

Summer Berry Shake

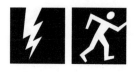

SERVES 1; MAKES ABOUT 2 CUPS

¹/₄ cup fresh or frozen **BLUEBERRIES**

¹/₄ cup fresh or frozen **RASPBERRIES**

5 large **STRAWBERRIES**, rinsed and trimmed, quartered

5 **ICE CUBES**, roughly broken

¹/₂ cup **CRANBERRY JUICE**

¹/₂ cup nonfat **STRAWBERRY** or **RASPBERRY FROZEN YOGURT** or **STRAWBERRY** or **RASPBERRY SORBET** (1 generous scoop)

Put the blueberries, raspberries, strawberries, ice cubes, cranberry juice, and yogurt in the canister of a blender. Blend until smooth. Serve immediately.

NUTRITIONAL ANALYSIS (per serving):
Total carbohydrates: 52 g / Protein: 6 g / Fat: .5 g / Dietary fiber: 5 g / Calories: 230

Mixed Fruit Shake

SERVES 1; MAKES ABOUT 2 CUPS

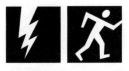

1/4 **BANANA** (about 1 1/2 inches)

2 fresh or frozen **STRAWBERRIES**, rinsed and trimmed if fresh, quartered

4 ounces fresh or canned **PINEAPPLE**, cored if fresh, cut into chunks

5 ounces **CANTALOUPE**, cut into chunks (about 1 cup)

5 ounces **HONEYDEW MELON**, cut into chunks (about 1 cup)

4 **ICE CUBES**, roughly broken

1/3 cup **APPLE JUICE**

Put the banana, strawberries, pineapple, cantaloupe, honeydew melon, ice cubes, and apple juice in the canister of a blender. Blend until smooth. Serve immediately.

NUTRITIONAL ANALYSIS (per serving):
Total carbohydrates: 46 g / Protein: 2 g / Fat: .5 g / Dietary fiber: 4 g / Calories: 180

Chocolate Whey Protein Shake

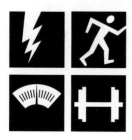

SERVES 1; MAKES ABOUT 2 CUPS

4 **STRAWBERRIES**, rinsed and trimmed, quartered

5 **ICE CUBES,** roughly broken

2/3 cup **APPLE JUICE**, **SKIM MILK**, or **WATER**

1 scoop **CHOCOLATE WHEY PROTEIN POWDER** (scant 1/3 cup), see Note

Put the strawberries, ice cubes, and apple juice in the canister of a blender. With the motor running, add the protein powder. Blend until smooth. Serve immediately.

NOTE: Protein powder makes shakes thick. You may have to stir the shake with a rubber spatula when partly blended and then continue blending.

NUTRITIONAL ANALYSIS (per serving):
Total carbohydrates: 27 g / Protein: 18.5 g / Fat: 1.5 g / Dietary fiber: 1.5 g / Calories: 190

The Pump Energy Shake

SERVES 1; MAKES ABOUT 2 CUPS

1 cup **SKIM MILK** or **RICE MILK**

6 **ICE CUBES**, roughly broken

1 scoop **SOURCE OF LIFE PROTEIN POWDER** (scant ¼ cup)

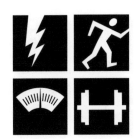

Put the milk and ice in the canister of a blender. With the motor running, add the protein powder. Blend until smooth. Serve immediately.

NUTRITIONAL ANALYSIS (with skim milk, per serving):
Total carbohydrates: 29 g / Protein: 22 g / Fat: 0 g / Dietary fiber: 1 g / Calories: 210

Banana-Strawberry Soy Protein Shake

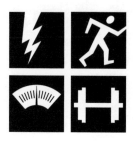

SERVES 1; MAKES ABOUT 2 CUPS

1/3 **BANANA** (about 2 inches long)

4 large **STRAWBERRIES**, rinsed and trimmed, quartered

8 **ICE CUBES**, roughly broken

1/4 cup **ORANGE JUICE**

1/2 cup **RICE MILK**

1 scoop **VANILLA SOY PROTEIN POWDER** (scant 1/4 cup), see Note

Put the banana, strawberries, ice cubes, orange juice, and rice milk in the canister of a blender. With the motor running, add the protein powder. Blend until smooth. Serve immediately.

NOTE: Protein powder makes shakes thick. You may have to stir the shake with a rubber spatula when partly blended and then continue blending.

NUTRITIONAL ANALYSIS (per serving):
Total carbohydrates: 46 g / Protein: 17 g / Fat: 1.5 g / Dietary fiber: 5 g / Calories: 260

Blueberry-Apple Protein Shake

SERVES 1; MAKES ABOUT 2 CUPS

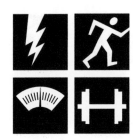

1/3 cup **BLUEBERRIES**

12 **ICE CUBES**, roughly broken

1 cup **APPLE JUICE**

1 scoop **VANILLA SOY PROTEIN POWDER** (scant 1/4 cup), see Note

Put the blueberries, ice cubes, and apple juice in the canister of a blender. With the motor running, add the protein powder. Blend until smooth. Serve immediately.

NOTE: Protein powder makes shakes thick. You may have to stir the shake with a rubber spatula when partly blended and then continue blending.

NUTRITIONAL ANALYSIS (per serving):

Total carbohydrates: 38 g / Protein: 18.5 g / Fat: 1.5 g / Dietary fiber: 1.5 g / Calories: 240

Creativity Juice

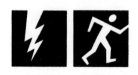

SERVES 2

1 **ROMAINE LETTUCE HEART**, roughly torn (7 to 8 cups)

4 ounces fresh **BABY SPINACH**

4 ribs **CELERY**, halved if necessary

One 6-inch-long **CUCUMBER**, halved if necessary

One ½-inch piece fresh **GINGER**

½ **LEMON**, cut into 2 wedges

Juice the lettuce, spinach, celery, cucumber, and ginger in a juice extractor. For ease, alternate the celery and cucumber with the leafy greens when putting the vegetables in the juice extractor. Garnish each glass with a lemon wedge and serve immediately.

NUTRITIONAL ANALYSIS (per serving):
Total carbohydrates: 17 g / Protein: 4 g / Fat: .5 g / Dietary fiber: 5 g / Calories: 70

Get-Up-and-Go Juice

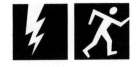

SERVES 2

3 medium **CARROTS**, halved if necessary
Two 6-inch-long **CUCUMBERS**, halved if
   necessary
1 medium **APPLE**, halved or quartered if
   necessary

1 medium **BEET**, thinly peeled, halved or
   quartered if necessary
One 1/2-inch piece fresh **GINGER**

Juice the carrots, cucumbers, apple, beet, and ginger in a juice extractor. Serve immediately.

NUTRITIONAL ANALYSIS (per serving):
Total carbohydrates: 31 g / Protein: 4 g / Fat: .5 g / Dietary fiber: 7 g / Calories: 140

Carrot-Apple-Celery Juice

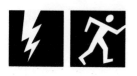

SERVES 2

4 medium **CARROTS**, halved if necessary

2 large **APPLES**, halved or quartered if
necessary

4 large ribs **CELERY**

Juice the carrots, apples, and celery in a juice extractor. Serve immediately.

NUTRITIONAL ANALYSIS (per serving):
Total carbohydrates: 48 g / Protein: 3 g / Fat: .5 g / Dietary fiber: 9 g / Calories: 190

Grapefruit-Orange Juice

SERVES 2

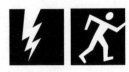

3 large **ORANGES**, peeled and halved
2 large **GRAPEFRUITS**, peeled and halved

¹/₂ **LEMON**, peeled

Juice the oranges, grapefruits, and lemon in a juice extractor. Serve immediately.

NUTRITIONAL ANALYSIS (per serving):
Total carbohydrates: 61 g / Protein: 5 g / Fat: .5 g / Dietary fiber: 11 g / Calories: 240

11.
Dressings and Sauces

Delicious Pesto Without Cheese / Soy Salad Dressing / Cucumber Yogurt Dressing / Oil and Vinegar Dressing with Herbs / Honey-Mustard Dressing / Mustard-Thyme Vinaigrette / Carrot-Ginger Dressing / Tahini Dressing

Delicious Pesto Without Cheese

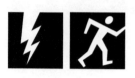

WE PROMISE YOU WON'T MISS THE CHEESE when you make this fresh-tasting pesto. We use it liberally on chicken and fish and in sandwiches in place of mayonnaise. There is also very little salt and not much oil—just good, clean flavor. Make a batch, keep it in the refrigerator, and eat it over two or three days.

MAKES ABOUT 1 1/2 CUPS

1/3 cup **PIGNOLI NUTS**
1 cup tightly packed **FRESH BASIL LEAVES**
1/3 cup **OLIVE OIL**

1/2 cup finely chopped **SWEET ONION**, such as Vidalia
1 tablespoon fresh **LEMON JUICE**

Preheat the oven to 350°F.

Spread the pignoli nuts on a baking sheet and roast for 6 to 8 minutes, stirring once or twice, until lightly browned and fragrant. Cool slightly.

In the bowl of a food processor fitted with the metal blade, combine the basil leaves, olive oil, onion, lemon juice, and pignoli nuts. Process until the consistency of chunky mayonnaise. Serve immediately or transfer to a glass container, cover the surface with plastic wrap, and refrigerate for up to 2 days.

NUTRITIONAL ANALYSIS (per 2-tablespoon serving):
Total carbohydrates: 2 g / Protein: 1 g / Fat: 9 g / Dietary fiber: 0 g / Calories: 90

Soy Salad Dressing

DRESSINGS MADE WITH SMOOTH, SILKEN TOFU are ultimately thick, satisfying, and healthful. This dressing is one of the very best, made with handfuls of fresh herbs and garden vegetables. Spoon it over steamed vegetables, on greens, and alongside broiled or pan-cooked chicken and fish. **MAKES ABOUT 1 1/2 CUPS**

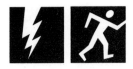

6 ounces **SOFT TOFU**

1 **KIRBY CUCUMBER**, peeled and coarsely chopped

1 **PLUM TOMATO**, chopped

1 **SHALLOT**, chopped

1/3 cup coarsely chopped **FRESH BASIL LEAVES**

3 tablespoons chopped **FRESH CILANTRO**

3 tablespoons fresh **LIME JUICE**

1 small clove **GARLIC**, minced, optional

Salt and freshly ground **BLACK PEPPER** to taste

Put all the ingredients in a blender and process until smooth. Use very soon after blending. This dressing does not store well.

NUTRITIONAL ANALYSIS (per 2-tablespoon serving):
Total carbohydrates: 1 g / Protein: 1 g / Fat: .5 g / Dietary fiber: 0 g / Calories: 10

Cucumber Yogurt Dressing

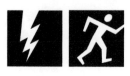

NOT SURPRISINGLY, WE LOVE TO SERVE THIS with grilled or roasted lamb, but it's also tasty with steamed and raw vegetables, such as salad greens. It keeps in the refrigerator for up to three days (which is as long as we like to keep anything in the fridge) and gives you a lot of flexibility when planning meals. Try this with baked tofu—you'll love it!

MAKES ABOUT 6 CUPS

1 cup nonfat **PLAIN YOGURT**
1/3 cup nonfat **SOUR CREAM**
1 cup loosely packed chopped **FRESH DILL**
Juice from 1/2 **LIME**
1 small clove **GARLIC**, finely minced

SEA SALT, optional
Freshly ground **BLACK PEPPER**, optional
4 medium **CUCUMBERS**, peeled and chopped
    into small cubes or wedges (about 5 cups)

In a mixing bowl, whisk together the yogurt, sour cream, dill, lime juice, and garlic. Add salt and pepper to taste, if desired.

Stir the cucumbers into the dressing.

NUTRITIONAL ANALYSIS (per 2-tablespoon serving):
Total carbohydrates: 1 g / Protein: 0 g / Fat: 0 g / Dietary fiber: 0 g / Calories: 5

Oil and Vinegar Dressing with Herbs

A SIMPLE OIL AND VINEGAR DRESSING BRINGS NEARLY ANY SALAD ALIVE, and this one is no exception. It's tangier than some because we don't use much oil. Since it requires so little oil, we suggest you use the best extra-virgin olive oil you have. Add the herbs we suggest or use your favorites. However you mix it, it's deliciously mysterious: What is that flavor? people will wonder. It's the herbs!

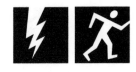

MAKES ABOUT 1 1/2 CUPS

1 cup **WHITE BALSAMIC VINEGAR**
1/2 cup fresh **LEMON JUICE**
2 tablespoons extra-virgin **OLIVE OIL**
2 teaspoons **DRIED BASIL**
1 teaspoon **DRIED THYME**

1/2 teaspoon **DRIED OREGANO**
1/4 teaspoon **DRIED MARJORAM**
1/4 teaspoon **CELERY SEED**
1/4 teaspoon **SEA SALT**, optional
Freshly ground **BLACK PEPPER**

In a small bowl, whisk together the vinegar, lemon juice, and olive oil. Add the basil, thyme, oregano, marjoram, and celery seed and whisk just until blended. Taste and add salt, if using, and pepper to taste.

Cover and set aside or refrigerate for at least 1 hour for the flavors to blend. Whisk before using. This will keep in the refrigerator for up to 3 days. Whisk before using.

NUTRITIONAL ANALYSIS (per 2-tablespoon serving):
Total carbohydrates: 4 g / Protein: 0 g / Fat: 2.5 g / Dietary fiber: 0 g / Calories: 40

Honey-Mustard Dressing

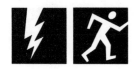

A GREAT, VERSATILE DRESSING. Our customers drizzle it over turkey burgers, steak burgers, and turkey breast, and it absolutely brings greens alive.

MAKES ABOUT 1/2 CUP

3 tablespoons **WATER** or **APPLE CIDER**

2 tablespoons **YELLOW MUSTARD**

1 1/2 teaspoons **HONEY**

1 tablespoon **APPLE CIDER VINEGAR**

1/8 teaspoon **CHINESE FIVE-SPICE POWDER**

Put all the ingredients in a blender and blend for a few seconds or until emulsified and smooth and the consistency of light cream. Use immediately.

NUTRITIONAL ANALYSIS (per 2-tablespoon serving):

Total carbohydrates: 2 g / Protein: 0 g / Fat: 0 g / Dietary fiber: 0 g / Calories: 10

Mustard-Thyme Vinaigrette

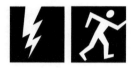

THINK BEYOND GREEN SALAD when you whisk up this dressing. As delicious as it is on a salad, it's also terrific drizzled over lean turkey breast, chicken, and steak.

MAKES ABOUT ½ CUP

1½ tablespoons extra-virgin **OLIVE OIL**

2 tablespoons fresh **LEMON JUICE**

2 tablespoons **WATER**

1 tablespoon roughly chopped **FRESH THYME**
    LEAVES

1 teaspoon grated **LEMON ZEST**

1 teaspoon **DIJON MUSTARD**

¼ teaspoon freshly ground **BLACK PEPPER**

In a small bowl, whisk together all the ingredients until blended. Serve immediately. You can cover and refrigerate the dressing for up to 2 days. Whisk before serving.

NUTRITIONAL ANALYSIS (per 2-tablespoon serving):
Total carbohydrates: 1 g / Protein: 0 g / Fat: 5 g / Dietary fiber: 0 g / Calories: 50

Carrot-Ginger Dressing

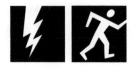

WE LOVE THIS DRESSING FOR ITS ASIAN FLAIR. It reminds us of the carrot-soy-based dressing you get in Japanese restaurants, but we like it even better! It doesn't have any oil, and with the lemon zest tastes light and fresh. We spoon this over green salad, steamed vegetables, baked tofu, and brown rice. It's endlessly versatile and keeps nicely for a few days in the refrigerator.

MAKES ABOUT 2 CUPS

One of the reasons I frequently purchase meals from [the Pump] is that I do not feel tired after a meal. I like to say if my meal does not drain energy from me, I am eating the right food. I really like the Tahini and Carrot-Ginger dressings. It is very difficult to find healthy, good-tasting dressings.
—MICHAEL RASHTI

3 cups **WATER**

2 **ONIONS**, coarsely chopped

2 medium **CARROTS**, peeled and coarsely chopped

2 tablespoons **APPLE CIDER VINEGAR**

2 teaspoons low-sodium **SOY SAUCE**

2 teaspoons shredded fresh **GINGER**

1/4 teaspoon grated **LEMON ZEST**

SEA SALT, optional

Put the water, onions, and carrots in a large saucepan. Bring to a boil over medium-high heat, reduce the heat to medium, and simmer, partially covered, for 20 to 30 minutes, or until the vegetables are very soft and you have about 1 1/4 cups of vegetables and liquid.

Remove the pan from the heat and let the vegetables cool in the liquid. Cover and refrigerate for at least 4 hours and up to 12 hours.

Pour the vegetables and cooking liquid in the canister of a blender. Add the vinegar, soy sauce, ginger, and lemon zest. Season with salt, if using. Blend until smooth. The dressing will be slightly thicker than heavy cream. Use immediately or cover and refrigerate for up to 3 days. Whisk before using.

NUTRITIONAL ANALYSIS (per 2-tablespoon serving):
Total carbohydrates: 3 g / Protein: 0 g / Fat: 0 g / Dietary fiber: 1 g / Calories: 15

Tahini Dressing

ELENA REALLY LOVES THIS DRESSING, which is why it's nearly always in our refrigerator. We spoon it over Baked Tofu, the Pump's Baked Falafel, and our Nature Burgers and love it for a lot of our Supercharged Plates. It dresses up plain brown rice, too. A real winner!

MAKES ABOUT 3 CUPS

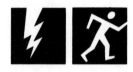

1 cup cooked **CANNELLINI BEANS**, page 107
1½ cups **WATER**
¼ cup **TAHINI**
¼ cup **WHITE WINE VINEGAR**
¼ cup fresh **LEMON JUICE**
2 teaspoons grated **LEMON ZEST**
¼ cup packed **FLAT-LEAF PARSLEY LEAVES**

1 small clove **GARLIC**, crushed, or 1 teaspoon **GARLIC POWDER**
1 small **SHALLOT**, minced
Pinch of **SEA SALT,** optional

Put all the ingredients except the shallot and salt in the canister of a blender and blend until smooth and the consistency of half-and-half. Stir in the shallot. Taste and season with salt. Serve immediately.

NUTRITIONAL ANALYSIS (per 2-tablespoon serving):
Total carbohydrates: 3 g / Protein: 1 g / Fat: 1.5 g / Dietary fiber: 1 g / Calories: 30

12.
Desserts

Baked Pineapple with Strawberry Sauce / Stewed Fruit with Orange Juice and Yogurt / Chocolate–Peanut Butter Protein Pudding / The Pump Pie Crust / Pump Apple Pie / Sweet Potato and Banana Pie / The Pump's Fruit Salad

Baked Pineapple with Strawberry Sauce

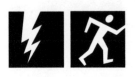

THIS STUNNING DESSERT IS MADE WITHOUT AN OUNCE OF FLOUR, cream, or butter. The first time you try it, you'll be blown away. We were! The sweeter the pineapple and the strawberries, the better the overall flavor, so look for ripe fruit.

SERVES 4

1 large firm, ripe **PINEAPPLE**, about 3½ pounds, see Variation

2 pints fresh **STRAWBERRIES**, washed, hulled, and sliced

⅓ cup **ORANGE JUICE** or **APPLE JUICE**

1 **CINNAMON STICK**, about 3 inches long

Preheat the oven to 375°F.

Peel pineapple and remove the core with a pineapple corer or a small, sharp knife. Discard the core. Slice the pineapple into rings or half moons (if it's easier) about ½ inch thick.

Combine the strawberries, juice, and cinnamon stick in a saucepan and bring to a boil over medium-high heat. Immediately reduce the heat and simmer for 20 to 25 minutes, or until the strawberries are soft. Remove and discard the cinnamon stick. Stir to blend. You will have about 1½ cups of sauce.

Meanwhile, lay the pineapple rings in a single layer on a nonstick baking sheet. Bake for 15 minutes. Turn the rings over and bake for 10 to 15 minutes longer or until the fruit is caramelized and lightly golden brown.

Arrange the pineapple rings on dessert plates and serve topped with the hot strawberry sauce.

VARIATION: You can substitute halved, peeled, and cored pears for the pineapple. You may find it easier to buy a peeled and cored pineapple, readily available in the produce department of most supermarkets.

NUTRITIONAL ANALYSIS (per serving):
Total carbohydrates: 30 g / Protein: 2 g / Fat: .5 g / Dietary fiber: 5 g / Calories: 120

Stewed Fruit with Orange Juice and Yogurt

MAKE THIS A FEW HOURS BEFORE YOU PLAN TO SERVE IT so that it has time to chill. The fruit stews to a sweet mass and the fruit-flavored yogurt brings all the flavors home. We like peach yogurt, but choose strawberry, raspberry, or another flavor if you prefer. You'll never be disappointed when this is dessert!

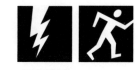

SERVES 4

2 pints fresh **STRAWBERRIES**, washed, hulled, and sliced

2 firm **APPLES** (about ³/₄ pound), peeled and chopped

¹/₂ cup fresh **ORANGE JUICE**

1 teaspoon finely grated **ORANGE ZEST**

1 teaspoon ground **CINNAMON**

2 **BANANAS**, sliced

One 8-ounce container **PEACH NONFAT YOGURT**

In a large saucepan, combine the strawberries, apples, orange juice, orange zest, and cinnamon. Cover, bring to a boil over medium heat, and immediately reduce the heat to medium low. Remove the cover and stir in the bananas.

Simmer gently, uncovered, for about 5 minutes, or until the fruit is soft.

Let cool for 10 to 15 minutes or refrigerate it until chilled. Spoon the fruit into 4 bowls and top each serving with yogurt.

NUTRITIONAL ANALYSIS (per serving):
Total carbohydrates: 44 g / Protein: 4 g / Fat: 1 g / Dietary fiber: 6 g / Calories: 180

Chocolate-Peanut Butter Protein Pudding

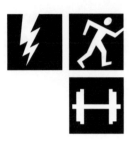

HAVE YOU NOTICED HOW MANY PROTEIN BARS in health food stores and supermarkets include chocolate and peanut butter? Here's the same combination but in a pudding you make yourself in a jiffy and then leave to chill for a few hours. You control the sweetness by making the right choice of peanut butter. We suggest natural peanut butter, which is as easy to find in supermarkets as the sugary variety. Eat this as dessert or a snack. Either way, you won't be disappointed!

SERVES 6

3 cups **SKIM MILK**
1 3-ounce package sugar-free cook-to-serve
    CHOCOLATE PUDDING MIX

2 scoops **CHOCOLATE WHEY PROTEIN**
    POWDER (scant 2/3 cup)
2 tablespoons natural creamy **PEANUT BUTTER**

In a large saucepan, whisk the milk and pudding mix together. Bring to a gentle simmer over medium-high heat, whisking constantly for 3 to 5 minutes until thickened. Do not let the milk boil.

Add the whey protein powder and peanut butter and whisk with a wire whisk until smooth.

Pour into six 6-ounce custard cups or ramekins. Set aside to cool and then refrigerate for 1 to 2 hours, or until well chilled.

NUTRITIONAL ANALYSIS (per serving):
Total carbohydrates: 21 g / Protein: 27 g / Fat: 3 g / Dietary fiber: 1 g / Calories: 220

The Pump Pie Crust

MOST PEOPLE THINK WE ARE NUTS when we tell them how we make this pie crust, but then they try it and bingo! It works! You have to treat it with care, as you do with all pastry dough, and it mustn't be too wet or too dry. You also must let it cool before you fill it. It's the most healthful pie crust we can imagine and tastes good, too. You'll never feel guilty when you eat this and you'll never feel cheated, either. Eating a poorly made pie with a fat-laden, production-line crust is unacceptable to us!

MAKES ONE 9-INCH SINGLE PIE CRUST

6 to 7 tablespoons **COLD RICE MILK**

1 tablespoon **ALMOND BUTTER**

1 cup whole wheat **PASTRY FLOUR**

1/2 teaspoon ground **CINNAMON**

Preheat the oven to 375°F.

In the bowl of a food processor fitted with the metal blade, combine 6 tablespoons of rice milk and the almond butter. Process until smooth.

Add the flour and cinnamon to the food processor and pulse 8 times or until the mixture is crumbly and moist. Add the remaining tablespoon of milk, if necessary.

Turn the dough out onto a generously floured surface, knead 6 to 8 times, or until cohesive, and pat into a smooth round. Using a rolling pin, gently roll the dough into a round about 10 inches in diameter. Lift the dough and drape it in a 9-inch pie plate. Gently press the dough over the bottom and up the sides of the pie plate. There won't be any overhang. If it's easier, pat the dough into a smooth circle and then drape in the pie plate and press into the pan.

NUTRITIONAL ANALYSIS (per serving):
Total carbohydrates: 26 g / Protein: 3 g / Fat: 1.5 g / Dietary fiber: 1 g / Calories: 140

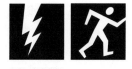

I always feel more energized after I eat the food and I never crash in the afternoon. I feel clean and healthy when I eat at the Pump. I have even gone down a dress size! It is just amazing to me that you can make your food so healthful and [still have it] taste so good. I've told all my friends and colleagues about it and even some personal trainers I know. I brought a bunch of your pies to Thanksgiving and no one could believe they were fat-free or how great they tasted.
—JESSICA TAYLOR, customer

Pump Apple Pie

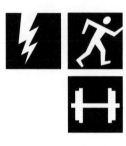

WE'RE WELL KNOWN FOR THIS PIE, AND ONCE YOU TASTE IT, we think you'll know why. No sugar but plenty of fruit and a little protein powder make it a rounded, balanced dish that can be served for dessert, a snack, or breakfast. It tastes of apples, pure and simple, and the granola gives enough crunchiness to turn it into a spectacular pie.

MAKES ONE 9-INCH PIE

1 **PUMP PIE CRUST**, page 181

2 firm **BAKING APPLES**, such as Granny Smith or Golden Delicious, peeled, cored, and sliced, see Note

2 softer **APPLES**, such as McIntosh, Ida Reds, or pippins, peeled, cored, and sliced, see Note

1 cup **APPLE CIDER**

1/4 cup **WATER**

1/2 teaspoon ground **CINNAMON**

2/3 cup **VANILLA WHEY POWDER**

2 teaspoons fresh **LEMON JUICE**, optional

1 teaspoon finely chopped **LEMON ZEST**, optional

1/3 cup old-fashioned **ROLLED OATS** (not instant)

3 tablespoons sliced **ALMONDS**

Preheat the oven to 375°F. with the rack in the lower third of the oven.

Bake the pie crust, already pressed into a shallow (standard) 9-inch pie plate, for about 5 minutes until dry to the touch. Cool on a wire rack while you prepare the filling. Do not turn off the oven unless you plan to finish the pie later.

In a large nonstick skillet, cook the apples, cider, and water and bring to a simmer over medium-high heat. Add the cinnamon, partially cover the skillet, and simmer for 6 to 7 minutes or until about half the apple slices begin to soften and appear translucent. The mixture will be juicy.

Remove the skillet from the heat and stir in the protein powder, lemon juice, and lemon zest, if using. Stir thoroughly with a rubber spatula to combine the ingredients without breaking the apples. Set aside to cool slightly.

Meanwhile, toast the topping by spreading the rolled oats and almonds in a shallow, 8- or 9-inch cake pan. Toast in the oven for 5 to 6 minutes or until lightly golden. Shake the pan a few times to insure even browning. Remove the topping from the oven and set aside.

Transfer the apple filling to the partially baked and cooled pie crust. Mound the filling slightly in the center of the crust. Top evenly with the rolled oat–almond topping.

Bake on the lowest rack of the oven for about 30 minutes, or until the filling is bubbling and the topping is golden brown.

Let the pie cool completely on a wire rack before serving. This will take at least 1 hour.

NOTE: The total weight of the apples, weighed together, should be about 1 3/4 pounds.

NUTRITIONAL ANALYSIS (per serving):
Total carbohydrates: 41.5 g / Protein: 8.5 g / Fat: 3.5 g / Dietary fiber: 3 g / Calories: 230

Sweet Potato and Banana Pie

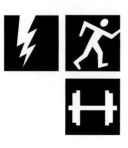

SWEET POTATOES ARE POWERHOUSES OF COMPLEX CARBOHYDRATES and bananas are great sources of potassium. We add protein powder to create the perfect pie, in terms of nutrition and flavor. If you work out, this is a pie for you! We add fresh lemon juice to keep the bananas from darkening as it sits at room temperature, but if you see a few flecks of brown, don't worry about them. They are harmless.

MAKES ONE 9-INCH PIE

1 1/2 pounds **SWEET POTATOES**, scrubbed but not peeled

1 **PUMP PIE CRUST**, page 181

2 1/2 ripe **BANANAS**, sliced and mashed

4 teaspoons freshly squeezed **LEMON JUICE**

1/2 cup **RICE MILK**

1/2 cup **VANILLA WHEY POWDER**

1/3 cup plus 1 tablespoon **EGG PROTEIN POWDER**, see Note

2 teaspoons **ALMOND BUTTER**, see Note

1 teaspoon ground **PUMPKIN PIE SPICE**, optional

Preheat the oven to 375°F.

With the tip of a sharp knife, pierce the potatoes in several places. Put in a shallow baking pan and bake for about 1 1/2 hours or until very tender when pierced with a fork. Remove from the oven.

Bake the pie crust, already pressed into a 9-inch deep-dish pie plate, for 6 to 8 minutes until dry to the touch. Cool on a wire rack while you prepare the filling. Turn off the oven.

Pick up each potato with a pot holder or tongs to prevent burning and carefully split in half. Set aside for about 1 hour to cool. When cool, scoop out the potato flesh. Discard the skin.

Preheat the oven to 375°F. again.

Put the mashed bananas and lemon juice in the bowl of an electric mixer and mix with a fork. Set aside for 15 minutes.

Add the cooled sweet potato flesh and, with the mixer on medium-high speed, beat until smooth with the paddle attachment. Add the rice milk, whey powder, egg protein powder, almond butter, and pumpkin pie spice, if using, and mix until incorporated. You will have about 4 cups of filling.

Spoon the sweet potato mixture into the prebaked pie shell and spread evenly. Bake for about 30 minutes or until the crust is lightly browned and the filling is set, puffed, and deep golden brown. The surface may split about the edges, which is fine.

Let the pie cool for 1 to 2 hours on a wire rack and serve at room temperature or slightly warm.

NOTE: Egg protein powder is not as easy to get as other protein powders and you may have to order it from a health food store. Almond butter is similar to peanut butter and is sold at health food stores.

NUTRITIONAL ANALYSIS (per serving):
Total carbohydrates: 26.5 g / Protein: 13.5 g / Fat: 2 g / Dietary fiber: 3 g / Calories: 170

The Pump's Fruit Salad

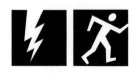

THE MELON IS THE KEY TO THIS FRUIT SALAD. Buy the honeydew and the cantaloupe a few days ahead of time and let them sit on the countertop for a few days to ripen. They will be fragrant and slightly soft at the stem end when ripe. (Believe us, underripe honeydew tastes like cucumber and won't do much for this salad.) The grapes and strawberries provide the sweetness. Just a little apple juice and scattering of cinnamon add indulgent flavor, although if you prefer, use mint instead of cinnamon.

SERVES 8

In a large bowl, combine the melon, pineapple, grapes, and strawberries.

4½ cups chunked **CANTALOUPE** (2¾-pound melon)

3 cups chunked **HONEYDEW MELON** (half a 3¾-pound melon)

3 cups chunked **PINEAPPLE** (8 ounces of peeled, cored pineapple)

1½ cups **SEEDLESS GREEN GRAPES**, stemmed

1½ cups **SEEDLESS RED GRAPES**, stemmed

1 cup rinsed, hulled, and quartered **STRAWBERRIES**

1 cup **APPLE JUICE**

1 teaspoon ground **CINNAMON** or 2 tablespoons sliced fresh **MINT LEAVES**

Add the apple juice and cinnamon or mint and toss gently to mix. Let the salad stand for 15 to 20 minutes for the flavors to blend, or refrigerate for up to 8 hours.

NOTE: For a less juicy fruit salad, omit the apple juice. Let the fruit stand for 15 to 20 minutes to release their juices.

You can substitute other fruits. Use crenshaw or another muskmelon. Other ideas include watermelon, kiwi, and star fruit.

NUTRITIONAL ANALYSIS (per serving):

Total carbohydrates: 42 g / Protein: 3 g / Fat: .5 g / Dietary fiber: 2 g / Calories: 170

As a fitness instructor, eating at the Pump gives me the energy I need to keep going throughout the day. My favorite meal at the Pump is the Baseball with a Crystal Light iced tea and an apple pie for dessert! I know I can rely on the Pump to give me "good for me" foods prepared in "good for me" ways. I know that they take my health seriously in every dish they make. Therefore, I also recommend it to my clients. Walk into the Pump and you'll see what I mean—the Pump's patrons are people who really care about their wellness, and we all know that we can put that in the hands of the Pump chefs each and every day! It is very important to nourish yourself—give your muscles TLC so they will be ready for their next challenge.

—DEBRA STROUGO, group fitness instructor at many New York City gyms
www.DebraFit.com

13.
Eggs and Pancakes

Mega Egg White Omelet / Pizzaiola Egg White Omelet / Turbo Chicken Omelet / The Pump's Spinach and Tomato Omelet / The Pump's Broccoli and Mozzarella Omelet / The Pump's Pepper and Mushroom Omelet / Elena's Spinach and Feta Omelet / Super-Balanced Baked Turkey Omelet / Steak-and-Egg Sandwich / Egg Delight Sandwich / Egg, Tofu, and Tomato Sandwich / The Pump's Protein Pancakes

Mega Egg White Omelet

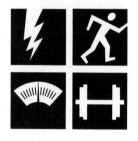

MAKE THIS OVERSIZE OMELET FOR THE WHOLE FAMILY. It's quick, delicious, and healthful. We add yellow bell peppers, but you could use red or orange peppers instead.
SERVES 2

12 large **EGG WHITES**
1 **SCALLION**, white part only, chopped
1/4 cup diced **YELLOW BELL PEPPER**
OLIVE OIL COOKING SPRAY

SEA SALT and freshly ground **BLACK PEPPER**, optional
KETCHUP, optional

Preheat the oven to 375°F.

Put the egg whites in a large bowl, and using a handheld electric mixer, whip until frothy. Stir in the scallion and bell pepper.

Spray a 9½-inch round glass dish or pie plate lightly with cooking spray. Pour the egg whites into the pan and bake for 18 to 20 minutes or until set and golden. Season to taste with salt and pepper.

Slide the omelet from the pan onto a serving plate. Slice and serve with ketchup, if desired.

NUTRITIONAL ANALYSIS (per serving):
Total carbohydrates: 3 g / Protein: 22 g / Fat: 1 g / Dietary fiber: 0 g / Calories: 120

Pizzaiola Egg White Omelet

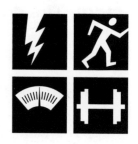

THIS TASTY OMELET DEFIES THE IDEA THAT EGG WHITE OMELETS ARE BORING! Make it as described here or if you have leftovers from Steak Pizzaiola on page 79, use them. Either way, what a great breakfast or lunch!

SERVES 1

1 large **PLUM TOMATO**, cored, seeded, and
   chopped (about ½ cup)
1 cup thinly sliced **WHITE** or **CREMINI**
   MUSHROOMS
3 tablespoons minced **RED BELL PEPPER**
½ teaspoon dried **BASIL**

⅛ teaspoon dried **OREGANO**
4 large **EGG WHITES**
OLIVE OIL COOKING SPRAY
SEA SALT and freshly ground **BLACK PEPPER**
   to taste, optional

In a medium nonstick skillet, cook the tomato, mushrooms, and pepper over low heat for 5 to 6 minutes until softened. Add the basil and oregano, stir to mix, and then remove the pan from the heat. Cover and set aside.

Whisk the egg whites until frothy.

Spray a medium nonstick skillet or large omelet pan with olive oil cooking spray and set it over medium heat. When hot, pour in the egg whites and cook until the egg whites are firm and lightly golden on the bottom. Using a large spatula, turn the omelet over in the pan and spoon the vegetables on top of the omelet. Season to taste with salt and pepper, if desired. Cook for 2 to 3 minutes longer, or until the omelet is set on the bottom. Slide from the pan onto a plate, folding the omelet over as you do.

NUTRITIONAL ANALYSIS (per serving):
Total carbohydrates: 15 g / Protein: 20 g / Fat: 2.5 g / Dietary fiber: 1 g / Calories: 160

The body needs a balance of carbs, proteins, and fats to function at its best. Those of us who live a very active lifestyle need to fuel our bodies with the best foods available. The Pump gives you just that. The complex carbs found in the brown rice, whole-wheat pita, and legumes will keep your gas tank full while the proteins and fats will help build the muscles you crave.

If I said I only had one favorite item it would be a lie. My mind changes with my appetite. In general I will eat a #88 Egg Delight sandwich two hours before I work out, or an energy shake 30 minutes before working out. After a good workout nothing beats #58, Lean & Mean, with lentils and hummus on top. It hits the spot, leaving me feeling pumped without being bloated. In general, you can't beat this food.

—JOEY SUAREZ, New York Police Department fitness trainer

Turbo Chicken Omelet

ALL OUR OMELETS ARE MADE WITH EGG WHITES, a terrific source of protein but without the cholesterol and fat of whole eggs. We call this the "turbo omelet" because of the double protein whammy: chicken and egg whites. We like asparagus tips with this, but you could use broccolini, broccoli florets, or spinach instead. Steve makes this omelet in the morning, puts it in the oven, and takes his shower. It's done when he is!

SERVES 1

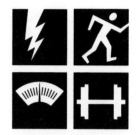

OLIVE OIL COOKING SPRAY

1 cup **ASPARAGUS** tips or coarsely chopped **BROCCOLINI**

5 to 6 ounces boneless, skinless **CHICKEN BREAST** or **TENDERS**

5 large **EGG WHITES**

¼ teaspoon freshly ground **BLACK PEPPER**

I live in Connecticut but go to the Pump every time I am in Manhattan. Your restaurant concept is phenomenal, as well as your food.
—STEVE SZABO

Preheat the oven to 400°F. Spray an ovenproof 8-inch nonstick skillet with olive oil cooking spray.

Put cold water in a saucepan to about a depth of 2 inches. Bring to a boil over medium-high heat. Add the asparagus tips or broccolini, reduce the heat to a simmer, and blanch for 1 minute. Drain and set aside to cool.

In a saucepan, bring 2 to 3 inches of water to a boil over medium-high heat. Add the chicken, reduce the heat to simmer, cover, and gently poach for 8 to 10 minutes, or until the chicken is pale-colored and cooked through. Alternatively, grill the chicken breast in a countertop grill until cooked through.

Let the chicken cool until you can handle it and then cut into chunks. You will have about 1 cup. (You can use leftover chicken here.)

Put the egg whites in a bowl and whisk until frothy. Add the chicken, blanched asparagus or broccolini, and pepper and stir to mix.

Pour the egg whites into the pan and bake for 8 to 10 minutes or until set.

NUTRITIONAL ANALYSIS (per serving):
Total carbohydrates: 7 g / Protein: 54 g / Fat: 5 g / Dietary fiber: 0 g / Calories: 290

The Pump's Spinach and Tomato Omelet

SPINACH AND TOMATOES ARE A LOVELY COMBINATION, and here they blend for a moist, tasty omelet—you won't miss cheese here!

SERVES 1

OLIVE OIL COOKING SPRAY
1 large **PLUM TOMATO**
5 large **EGG WHITES**

1 cup loosely packed fresh **BABY SPINACH LEAVES**, washed, dried, and chopped
½ teaspoon fresh **THYME LEAVES**

Preheat the oven to 400°F. Spray an ovenproof 8-inch nonstick skillet with cooking spray.

Halve the tomato, gently squeeze out the seeds, and cut into small dice. Pat dry with a paper towel to absorb as much excess moisture as possible. You will have about ½ cup of diced tomato.

In a mixing bowl, whisk the egg whites until frothy. Add the tomato, spinach, and thyme and mix gently. Pour into the pan and bake for 15 to 20 minutes or until set and lightly golden.

NUTRITIONAL ANALYSIS (per serving):
Total carbohydrates: 7 g / Protein: 19 g / Fat: 2 g / Dietary fiber: 2 g / Calories: 120

The Pump's Broccoli and Mozzarella Omelet

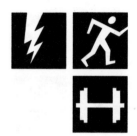

ALTHOUGH THERE IS NOT A LOT OF CHEESE, when you're in the mood for a cheese omelet, this one fits the bill. These omelets are good places to try soy cheese if you haven't integrated it into your diet. We love it with broccoli, but you could substitute asparagus tips or spinach.

SERVES 1

OLIVE OIL COOKING SPRAY

4 **BROCCOLI** florets

5 large **EGG WHITES**

1/4 teaspoon dried, crumbled **MARJORAM LEAVES**

2 ounces shredded nonfat **MOZZARELLA** or **SOY CHEESE**

Preheat the oven to 400°F. Spray an ovenproof 8-inch-square nonstick pan with nonstick cooking spray.

Put cold water in a saucepan to about a depth of 2 inches. Bring to a boil over medium-high heat. Add the broccoli florets, reduce the heat to a simmer, and blanch for 1 minute. Drain, set aside to cool, and slice into thin pieces.

In a mixing bowl, whisk the egg whites until frothy. Add the broccoli florets and marjoram and stir gently to mix.

Pour the egg whites into the pan and bake for 8 minutes or until the eggs are nearly set. Sprinkle with the cheese and return to the oven for 1 to 2 minutes or until the cheese melts and the top is lightly golden.

NUTRITIONAL ANALYSIS (per serving):
Total carbohydrates: 6 g / Protein: 38 g / Fat: 2 g / Dietary fiber: 2 g / Calories: 190

The Pump's Pepper and Mushroom Omelet

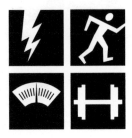

STEVE LOVES MUSHROOMS FOR THEIR RICH, EARTHY FLAVOR and luscious texture, and here they blend nicely with red bell peppers and shallots. If you feel ambitious, cook the vegetables in a nonstick pan for a few minutes before mixing them with the egg whites to deepen their flavors, but this step is not necessary.

SERVES 1

OLIVE OIL COOKING SPRAY
5 **EGG WHITES**
1/4 cup diced **RED BELL PEPPER**

3 tablespoons minced **SHALLOTS**
1/2 cup sliced **CREMINI** or **WHITE MUSHROOMS** (about 1 1/2 ounces)

Preheat the oven to 400°F. Spray an ovenproof 8-inch nonstick skillet with nonstick cooking spray.

In a mixing bowl, whisk the egg whites until frothy. Add the pepper, shallots, and mushrooms and stir gently to mix.

Pour the egg whites into the pan and bake for 8 to 10 minutes or until set and lightly golden.

NUTRITIONAL ANALYSIS (per serving):
Total carbohydrates: 10 g / Protein: 20 g / Fat: 2 g / Dietary fiber: 0 g / Calories: 140

Elena's Spinach and Feta Omelet

WE MAKE THIS OMELET FOR A WEEKEND BREAKFAST OR BRUNCH. It's a heavenly combination of spinach and feta. We make it with dried oregano, but if you wanted to try another herb, go for it!

SERVES 1

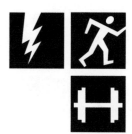

OLIVE OIL COOKING SPRAY

5 large **EGG WHITES**

2 cups loosely packed fresh **BABY SPINACH**, washed, dried and chopped

3 ounces low-fat **FETA,** crumbled (about 2/3 cup)

1/2 teaspoon crumbled dried **OREGANO**

1/4 teaspoon freshly ground **BLACK PEPPER**, optional

Preheat the oven to 400°F. Spray an ovenproof 8-inch skillet with nonstick cooking spray.

In a mixing bowl, whisk the egg whites until frothy. Add the spinach, feta, oregano, and pepper, if desired, and stir gently to mix.

Pour the egg whites into the pan and bake for 8 to 10 minutes or until set and lightly golden.

NUTRITIONAL ANALYSIS (per serving):

Total carbohydrates: 10 g / Protein: 37 g / Fat: 11 g / Dietary fiber: 3 g / Calories: 270

Super-Balanced Baked Turkey Omelet

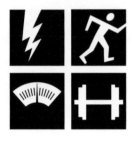

DO YOUR MUSCLES A FAVOR and eat this an hour or two after working out. It's filling but has very little fat or cholesterol and is a terrific source of protein.

SERVES 1

5 ounces chopped **TURKEY BREAST**
OLIVE OIL COOKING SPRAY
5 large **EGG WHITES**
2 ounces fresh **SPINACH LEAVES**, washed, dried, and chopped (about 2 cups)

1 teaspoon **FRESH THYME LEAVES**
¼ teaspoon freshly ground **BLACK PEPPER**
2 whole wheat **PITA BREADS**, optional
3 tablespoons **VEGETARIAN CHILI**, page 99 or **LENTIL SOUP**, page 29

Preheat the oven to 400°F. or preheat a countertop grill, such as a George Foreman Grill. Form the turkey into a patty about ½ inch thick.

In a nonstick skillet or on the grill, cook the turkey burger for 8 to 9 minutes, turning once, over medium-high heat until cooked through.

Meanwhile, in a mixing bowl, whisk the egg whites until frothy.

Spray an ovenproof 8- or 9-inch nonstick skillet with nonstick cooking spray.

Chop the burger into pieces and add to the egg whites with the spinach leaves, thyme, and pepper. Stir gently and pour into the ovenproof skillet. Bake for 8 to 10 minutes or until the eggs are set.

Slice the top off the pita breads, if using. Put the bread in the oven for about 30 seconds or just until warm.

Serve the omelet with the chili or lentil soup spooned over the top. Or spoon the cooked egg into the pita pocket, top with chili or lentil soup, and serve.

NUTRITIONAL ANALYSIS (per serving):
Total carbohydrates: 12 g / Protein: 63 g / Fat: 3 g / Dietary fiber: 4 g / Calories: 330

Steak-and-Egg Sandwich

EAT THIS HIGH-PROTEIN SANDWICH for breakfast or lunch. You will be totally satisfied, plus have all the energy you need.

SERVES 1

OLIVE OIL COOKING SPRAY

6 ounces lean **CHOPPED SIRLOIN**

1/2 cup diced **ONIONS**

1/2 teaspoon chopped fresh **ROSEMARY LEAVES**

1/4 teaspoon freshly ground **BLACK PEPPER**

5 large **EGG WHITES**

1 whole wheat 7-inch **PITA BREAD**

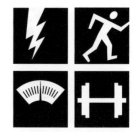

Preheat the oven to 400°F. Spray an ovenproof 8- or 9-inch nonstick skillet with cooking spray.

Cook the meat in the skillet over medium-high heat for about 2 minutes, stirring to break up the meat. Add the onions, rosemary, and pepper. Cook for 2 to 3 minutes longer until the onions soften and the meat browns. Drain off any fat and set aside for about 5 minutes to cool.

Meanwhile, in a mixing bowl, whisk the egg whites until frothy. Add the meat mixture and stir gently to mix.

Return the mixture to the skillet. Bake for 8 to 10 minutes or until the eggs are set.

Slice the top off the pita pocket. Put the bread in the oven for about 30 seconds or just until warm. Using tongs or a slender spatula, layer the cooked egg in the pita pocket and serve.

NUTRITIONAL ANALYSIS (per serving):
Total carbohydrates: 30 g / Protein: 56 g / Fat: 11 g / Dietary fiber: 5 g / Calories: 440

> The Pump does not have fried food and they do not use butter, bacon, egg yolks, sugar, white bread, oil, or salt in their food preparation. They emphasize protein and vegetables and don't stray from those commitments. For this reason I feel confident in patronizing The Pump.
> —JACQUELINE LAVALLE, Customer

Egg Delight Sandwich

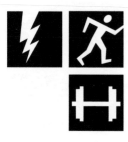

THIS VEGETARIAN SANDWICH IS GREAT FOR BRUNCH OR LUNCH. We love it with the broccoli and cheese, and if you want to add tomatoes, go for it.

SERVES 1

OLIVE OIL COOKING SPRAY
3 **BROCCOLI** florets
5 large **EGG WHITES**
2 to 3 **SCALLIONS**, green parts only, thinly sliced

2½ ounces shredded nonfat **MOZZARELLA** (about ½ cup)
Freshly ground **BLACK PEPPER**, optional
1 whole wheat 7-inch **PITA BREAD**, toasted, optional

Preheat the oven to 400°F. Spray an ovenproof 8-inch nonstick skillet with cooking spray.

Put cold water in a saucepan to about a depth of 2 inches. Bring to a boil over medium-high heat. Add the broccoli, reduce the heat to a simmer, and blanch for 1 minute. Drain and set aside to cool. Cut into thin slices.

In a mixing bowl, whisk the egg whites until frothy. Add the scallions and sliced broccoli and stir gently to mix.

Pour the egg whites into the pan and bake for 8 to 10 minutes or until the eggs are nearly set. Sprinkle with the cheese and return to the oven for about 2 minutes or until the cheese melts and the top is lightly golden. Season with pepper, if desired.

Serve plain or stuffed into the pita pocket, if desired.

NUTRITIONAL ANALYSIS (per serving):
Total carbohydrates: 32 g / Protein: 42 g / Fat: 3 g / Dietary fiber: 6 g / Calories: 320

Egg, Tofu, and Tomato Sandwich

THIS IS ONE OF OUR FAVORITES because of the protein hit from both the egg whites and the tofu. Non-vegetarians like it, too.

SERVES 1

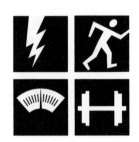

OLIVE OIL COOKING SPRAY
3 **BROCCOLI** florets, halved
3 ounces firm **TOFU**, diced
1/3 cup diced **TOMATO**

2 tablespoons minced **CHIVES**
5 large **EGG WHITES**
1 whole wheat 7-inch **PITA BREAD**, toasted, optional

Preheat the oven to 400°F. Spray an ovenproof 8-inch nonstick skillet with nonstick cooking spray.

Put cold water in a saucepan to about a depth of 2 inches. Bring to a boil over medium-high heat. Add the broccoli, reduce the heat to a simmer, and blanch for 1 minute. Drain and set aside to cool. Cut into slices.

In a small bowl, toss the broccoli with the tofu, tomato, and chives.

In a mixing bowl, whisk the egg whites until frothy. Lift the vegetables from the bowl with a slotted spoon to drain. Add to the eggs and mix gently. Pour into the pan and bake for 10 to 12 minutes or until set and lightly golden.

Serve plain or stuffed into the pita pocket, if desired.

NUTRITIONAL ANALYSIS (per serving):
Total carbohydrates: 35 g / Protein: 35 g / Fat: 9 g / Dietary fiber: 8 g / Calories: 340

The Pump's Protein Pancakes

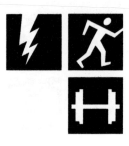

THESE ARE NOT REGULAR BREAKFAST PANCAKES but instead are a blending of protein and carbohydrates that produces a balanced meal. These are great for dieters as a once-a-week treat, but for bodybuilders, they are terrific. We have customers who like these alongside eggs—that's how good they are for building muscle.

SERVES 4; MAKES 8 TO 10 PANCAKES

6 heaping tablespoons **MULTIGRAIN PANCAKE MIX** (about 3 ounces), see Note

5 large **EGG WHITES**

1/2 cup **SKIM MILK**

3 scoops of **WHEY PROTEIN POWDER** (about 1 scant cup)

VEGETABLE COOKING SPRAY

2 cups sliced **BANANAS**, **BLUEBERRIES**, or sliced **STRAWBERRIES**, or **MIXED FRUIT**, optional

Preheat the oven to 375°F.

In a bowl, whisk together the pancake mix, egg whites, milk, and protein powder. When smooth, set aside to stand for 10 minutes so the batter can thicken.

Spray 2 nonstick baking sheets with vegetable oil spray. Make pancakes, using a scant 1/4 cup of pancake batter for each one. Using a light hand, top the pancakes with fruit, if desired, and bake for 5 to 7 minutes or until lightly browned around the edges and cooked through in the center. Do not overcook or they will toughen. Flip the pancakes over onto plates and serve hot with more fruit, if desired.

NOTE: Multigrain pancake mix is easily available in health food stores. The pancakes don't puff up like other pancakes do.

NUTRITIONAL ANALYSIS (per serving):

Total carbohydrates: 18.5 g / Protein: 21 g / Fat: 1.5 g / Dietary fiber: 2 g / Calories: 175

COOKING EGG WHITES

Whisk 5 large egg whites in a small bowl with a fork.

Pour the whites into a small baking dish that has been sprayed

with cooking spray. Bake in a preheated 400°F oven for 8 to

10 minutes or until set. Five whites is enough for one serving,

depending on how hungry you are!

14.
Snacks

Quick Tuna Fix / Hot Zucchini Strips with Shallots / Rice Cakes with Banana / Rice Cakes with Fruity Cottage Cheese / Rice Cake Cereal Snack / Blueberries and Strawberries with Yogurt / Frozen Yogurt with Protein

Quick Tuna Fix

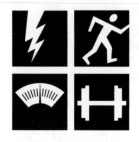

WHEN YOU'RE A LITTLE HUNGRY, THIS SNACK HITS THE SPOT. If you're a little hungrier than usual, spread it over rice cakes. There's no mayonnaise in this tuna salad, which we think makes it lighter and more interesting.

SERVES 2

One 6-ounce can **WHITE** or **ALBACORE TUNA**, packed in water, drained well
2 ribs **CELERY**, finely chopped
1 small **ONION**, minced
¼ cup minced flat-leaf **PARSLEY LEAVES**

¼ cup **WHITE BALSAMIC VINEGAR**
2 tablespoons fresh **LEMON JUICE**
1 tablespoon extra-virgin **OLIVE OIL**
4 **RICE CAKES**, optional

Put the drained tuna in a mixing bowl and flake it with a fork. Add the celery, onion, parsley, vinegar, lemon juice, and olive oil. Mix well. Serve spooned on rice cakes, if you want.

NUTRITIONAL ANALYSIS (per serving):
Total carbohydrates: 11 g / Protein: 21 g / Fat: 5 g / Dietary fiber: 1 g / Calories: 170

Hot Zucchini Strips with Shallots

THIS HEALTHFUL SNACK CAN DOUBLE AS A SIDE DISH. Mild zucchini strips are baked on a bed of aromatic shallots for a lovely flavor that makes them hard to resist.
SERVES 4

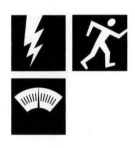

OLIVE OIL COOKING SPRAY

2 large **SHALLOTS**, peeled, thinly sliced and separated into rings (about 1 cup)

4 medium **ZUCCHINI**, ends trimmed and thinly sliced lengthwise

½ cup chopped flat-leaf **PARSLEY**

SEA SALT, optional

Preheat the oven to 375°F. Spray 2 shallow baking pans with olive oil cooking spray.

Spread the shallots in both pans, dividing them evenly. Top with the zucchini slices and spray lightly with cooking spray. Bake for 15 to 20 minutes or until they begin to soften. Turn the slices over and sprinkle with parsley. Bake for 12 to 15 minutes longer or until the zucchini is cooked through and tender. (For slightly crispy zucchini, leave the pans in the turned-off hot oven for about 15 minutes.) Serve hot from the oven, seasoned with salt, if desired.

NUTRITIONAL ANALYSIS (per serving):
Total carbohydrates: 8 g / Protein: 2 g / Fat: .5 g / Dietary fiber: 1 g / Calories: 35

Rice Cakes with Banana

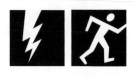 **WE CONFESS THAT IT TOOK A WHILE FOR BOTH OF US TO "MAKE FRIENDS"** with rice cakes, but now we happily eat them all the time. When Steve was on a strict weight-reducing diet, he ate them topped with fruit to satisfy any cravings for sweets. Rice cakes quell hunger pangs and help you avoid junk food. Make sure the bananas are very ripe and soft.

SERVES 6

2 ripe **BANANAS**
4 tablespoons **ALL-FRUIT JAM**, such as
   blueberry, strawberry, or raspberry

2/3 cup **VANILLA** or **CHOCOLATE WHEY**
   PROTEIN POWDER
6 plain or multigrain salt-free **RICE CAKES**

In a bowl, mash the bananas with a fork. Mix in the jam and the whey protein. Spread the mixture on the rice cakes and serve.

NUTRITIONAL ANALYSIS (per serving):
Total carbohydrates: 23 g / Protein: 25 g / Fat: .5 g / Dietary fiber: 1 g / Calories: 200

Rice Cakes with Fruity Cottage Cheese

COTTAGE CHEESE MIXED WITH FRUIT JAM tastes like cheesecake to us. Of course, this snack is far better for your overall health, and the protein powder boosts its benefits.

SERVES 8

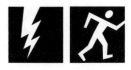

2 cups nonfat **COTTAGE CHEESE**

4 tablespoons **ALL-FRUIT JAM**, such as blueberry, strawberry, or raspberry

1/2 cup **SOY PROTEIN POWDER**, such as Spirutein

8 plain or multigrain salt-free **RICE CAKES**

In a bowl, stir together the cottage cheese and jam. Mix in the protein powder. Spread the mixture on the rice cakes and serve.

NUTRITIONAL ANALYSIS (per serving):

Total carbohydrates: 24 g / Protein: 17 g / Fat: 1 g / Dietary fiber: 0g / Calories: 180

Rice Cake
Cereal Snack

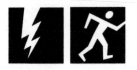

IF YOU EAT THIS IN THE MORNING FOR BREAKFAST, you won't feel hungry until lunch, and if you indulge in the mid-afternoon, you won't be tempted to snack on less healthful foods before dinner. **SERVES 2**

I have eaten lunch almost exclusively at the Pump for well over two years now. I lost about thirty pounds and have recommended the Pump to countless friends. My friends have done the same.
—ANTHONY TORSIELLO, customer

4 plain or multigrain salt-free **RICE CAKES**
1/2 cup **RAISINS**

1 1/3 cups **SKIM**, **SOY**, or **RICE MILK**

In a cereal bowl, crumble 2 rice cakes. Add half the raisins and half the skim milk. Stir and serve. Repeat with the remaining ingredients to make another serving.

NUTRITIONAL ANALYSIS (per serving):
Total carbohydrates: 55 g / Protein: 9 g / Fat: .5 g / Dietary fiber: 3 g / Calories: 260

Blueberries and Strawberries with Yogurt

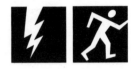

NOTHING COULD BE EASIER OR MORE DELICIOUS THAN THIS SNACK. If you have the berries rinsed, sliced, and waiting in the fridge, spoon some yogurt over them anytime you have a craving for a yummy, quick fix. The mint perks up the flavor as nothing else can!

SERVES 4

2 cups washed, stemmed, and sliced **STRAW-BERRIES**

1 cup **BLUEBERRIES**, stems removed, rinsed

2 cups nonfat **PLAIN YOGURT**

2 tablespoons fresh chopped **MINT**, optional, for garnish

In a large bowl, mix together the strawberries and blueberries.

Spoon the yogurt into 4 small bowls. Divide the berries evenly between the bowls, stir gently, and serve.

NUTRITIONAL ANALYSIS (per serving):

Total carbohydrates: 21 g / Protein: 6 g / Fat: .5 g / Dietary fiber: 3 g / Calories: 100

Frozen Yogurt with Protein

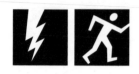

ONE NIGHT AFTER WORKING OUT AT THE GYM, Steve sprinkled some protein powder over frozen yogurt and discovered a favorite snack! It provides good energy and tastes like a frosty pudding, so it's a sweet treat, too. And it couldn't be easier.

SERVES 2

1 cup nonfat **VANILLA** or **COFFEE FROZEN YOGURT**

¼ cup **CHOCOLATE** or **VANILLA PROTEIN POWDER** (1 generous scoop)

¼ teaspoon **ESPRESSO POWDER**, optional

Scoop the yogurt into a bowl and let it sit at room temperature for about 5 minutes to soften just slightly.

Sprinkle with protein powder and espresso powder, if using, and stir to mix. Eat immediately.

NUTRITIONAL ANALYSIS (per serving):
Total carbohydrates: 19 g / Protein: 17 g / Fat: 0 g / Dietary fiber: 1 g / Calories: 150

For the other 23 hours that I'm not with my clients, it's essential for them to establish awareness and control of what they put into their bodies. The Pump assists by offering the other key component that I do not have full monitoring over . . . proper food intake. I rest a little easier now when my clients leave, knowing they are going to eat at the Pump.

My best advice? Teach yourself some form of self-discipline or control, and start with how you treat your body and what you put in it. Nourish it, water it, exercise it . . . earn that body you want! And be thankful for it. Remember, you control your environment—your environment doesn't control you.

—GREGG MIELE, New York City Strength and Conditioning Industries
www.Self-Discipline.com

15.
Super-
charged
Plates

Muscle Power Plate / Lean and Mean Plate / Champion Plate / Lean Body Plate / Diesel Plate / Dionysus Plate / The Rock Plate / Easy Rider Plate / Flying High Plate / Gigante Plate

Muscle Power Plate

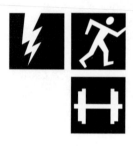

WE OFTEN THINK OF THE FAMOUS CARTOON SAILOR POPEYE, whose strength was maintained by his love of spinach, but this supercharged plate is also for the tahini lovers in the crowd. It's great for lunch or dinner, but we suggest replacing the brown rice with steamed vegetables if you eat this for supper.

SERVES 1

½ cup cooked **BROWN RICE**, page 139
½ cup steamed **SPINACH**, page 138
1 serving **GRILLED LEMON CHICKEN**, sliced,
    page 91

¼ cup **TAHINI DRESSING**, page 175

Preheat the oven to 375°F.

Spread the rice in a shallow baking dish (a pie plate works well). Spread the steamed spinach over the rice and top with the sliced chicken. Spoon the tahini evenly over the chicken. Bake for about 10 minutes or until heated through. Serve immediately.

NUTRITIONAL ANALYSIS (per serving):
Total carbohydrates: 38 g / Protein: 42 g / Fat: 12 g / Dietary fiber: 6 g / Calories: 410

Lean and Mean Plate

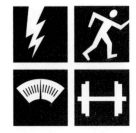

FOR EVERYONE LIFTING WEIGHTS AND WORKING OUT with an eye toward being ripped, this protein-rich supercharged plate wakes up your muscles. We know bodybuilders who order this a day or two before a competition. It fills you up and you'll never feel weak after eating this combination of foods. This plate is delicious topped with lentil soup.

SERVES 1

1 serving **STEAMED GREEN AND WHITE VEGETABLES**, page 124

1 serving **GRILLED LEMON CHICKEN**, sliced, page 91

¼ cup **MUSTARD-THYME VINAIGRETTE**, page 173, optional

Preheat the oven to 375°F.

Spread the vegetables in a shallow baking dish (a pie plate works well). Top with the sliced chicken and spoon the dressing, if using, evenly over the chicken. Bake for about 10 minutes or until heated through. Serve immediately.

NUTRITIONAL ANALYSIS (per serving):
Total carbohydrates: 14 g / Protein: 38 g / Fat: 4 g / Dietary fiber: 5 g / Calories: 230

Champion Plate

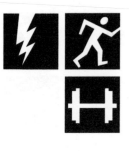

THE COMBINATION OF BROWN RICE, STEAMED VEGETABLES, AND CHICKEN is the perfect meal. Eat it for lunch for a high level of energy for the rest of the day. You are what you eat!
SERVES 1

½ cup cooked **BROWN RICE**, page 139
1 serving **STEAMED GREEN** and **WHITE VEGETABLES**, page 124
1 serving **MARINATED ROSEMARY-GARLIC CHICKEN**, sliced, page 88

3 tablespoons **CARROT-GINGER DRESSING**, page 174, optional

Preheat the oven to 375°F.

Spread the rice in a shallow baking dish (a pie plate works well). Spread the steamed vegetables over the rice and top with the sliced chicken. Drizzle the dressing, if using, over the chicken. Bake for about 10 minutes or until heated through. Serve immediately.

NUTRITIONAL ANALYSIS (per serving):
Total carbohydrates: 36 g / Protein: 40 g / Fat: 4.5 g / Dietary fiber: 7 g / Calories: 330

Lean Body Plate

THIS FILLING MEAL IS GREAT FOR ANYONE looking to lose body fat and build muscle. We love the flavor of the chili paired with the spinach and tempered by the simple baked chicken.

SERVES 1

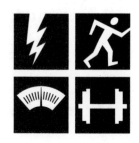

OLIVE OIL COOKING SPRAY

1 boneless, skinless **CHICKEN BREAST**, 5 to 6 ounces

½ cup hot steamed **SPINACH**, page 138

1 teaspoon chopped **RED BELL PEPPER**

1 teaspoon minced **ONION**

½ cup hot **VEGETARIAN CHILI**, page 99

Preheat the oven to 400°F.

Spray a small shallow baking pan with olive oil cooking spray. Lay the chicken in the pan and bake for 8 minutes or until cooked through. Remove from the pan. When cool enough, slice into strips.

Spread the spinach in a deep plate or shallow bowl and top with the sliced chicken. Sprinkle the pepper and onion over the chicken. Pour the chili over the top and serve immediately.

NUTRITIONAL ANALYSIS (per serving):

Total carbohydrates: 15 g / Protein: 38 g / Fat: 6 g / Dietary fiber: 5 g / Calories: 250

Nothing is more important than your health and taking care of your mind and body. Your body performs to its greatest potential when it is well fueled. The Pump has made every effort to ensure the nutrition part of your lifestyle meets the highest standards.

—ANTHONY CARILLO

My favorite menu item is the **Lean and Mean Supercharged Plate** with the extra scoop of lentil soup. This dish is an excellent source of protein, combining the chicken and lentils, with fresh steamed vegetables for carbohydrate, and is delicious!

It is always important to bring positive energy to all that you do. In the fitness business I try my best to help people reach their goals—making them healthier, stronger and more positive. The Pump offers people the chance to eat healthy and enjoy the variety in their food choices.

—AMY STODDARD

Anthony and Amy are fitness instructors at Iron Yoga
www.ironyoga.com

Diesel Plate

BUILDING MUSCLE? TRY THIS PLATE. We promise you will have enough energy after eating this plate full of flavor and protein to bench-press hundreds of pounds! You will have energy all day.
SERVES 1

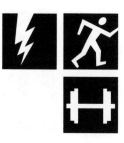

½ cup hot cooked **BROWN RICE**, page 139
1 serving hot **GRILLED LEMON CHICKEN**,
    sliced, page 91

½ cup hot **VEGETARIAN CHILI**, page 99

In a deep plate or shallow bowl, spread the brown rice in an even layer. Top with the chicken slices. Spoon the chili over the chicken and serve immediately.

NUTRITIONAL ANALYSIS (per serving):
Total carbohydrates: 36 g / Protein: 38 g / Fat: 5 g / Dietary fiber: 5 g / Calories: 330

The Diesel Supercharged Plate is by far my most favorite [menu item] at the Pump. After a grueling workout at the gym, the only thing on my mind is to fuel my body back up. How appropriately named is the Diesel?
—T. LEE, customer

Dionysus Plate

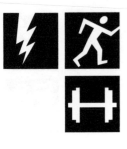

CHICKEN MIXED WITH CUCUMBER, TOMATOES, AND ONIONS blends perfectly with our never-fail pasta. You could make this plate with rice, if you prefer, or substitute steamed spinach or broccoli for the pasta. It's an outstanding meal.

SERVES 1

OLIVE OIL COOKING SPRAY

1 skinless, boneless **CHICKEN BREAST**, 5 to 6 ounces

3 tablespoons finely chopped **CUCUMBER**

2 tablespoons finely chopped **TOMATO**

1 tablespoon minced **ONION**

¼ cup **TAHINI DRESSING**, page 175

2 tablespoons **SOY SAUCE**

1 tablespoon **HOT PEPPER SAUCE**, optional

2 ounces whole wheat **FETTUCCINE** or **SPAGHETTI**

Preheat the oven to 400°F.

Spray a small shallow baking pan with olive oil cooking spray. Lay the chicken in the pan and bake for 6 minutes or until nearly cooked through. Remove from the pan but do not turn off the oven. When cool enough, slice the chicken into strips.

Return the chicken to the pan and add the cucumber, tomato, and onion. Toss to mix.

Spoon the dressing over the chicken and vegetables and add the soy sauce and hot sauce, if desired. Bake for 10 to 12 minutes or until the chicken is thoroughly cooked, the vegetables are soft, and the sauce is bubbling hot.

Meanwhile, cook the pasta in a saucepan of rapidly boiling water for about 8 minutes or until al dente. Drain.

Put the pasta on a plate and top with the chicken mixture. Serve immediately.

NUTRITIONAL ANALYSIS (per serving):
Total carbohydrates: 53 g / Protein: 46 g / Fat: 13 g / Dietary fiber: 5 g / Calories: 500

The Rock Plate

WE CAME UP WITH THIS PLATE WHEN STEVE REMEMBERED TRAINING years ago with a trainer from the old school. He insisted Steve eat only brown rice, tuna, and broccoli for two weeks while he worked out with weights. It worked! We spoon some soup over the supercharged plate to add another flavor dimension.

SERVES 1

½ cup hot cooked **BROWN RICE**, page 139

1 serving hot **STEAMED GREEN AND WHITE VEGETABLES**, page 124, see Note

One 6-ounce can water-packed **ALBACORE TUNA**, drained and flaked with a fork

1½ cups hot **CARROT-SWEET POTATO SOUP**, page 28

1 to 2 tablespoons fresh **LEMON JUICE**

In a deep plate or shallow bowl, spread the brown rice in an even layer. Top with the steamed vegetables and tuna. Pour the soup over the tuna and season with the lemon juice. Serve immediately.

NOTE: You can substitute steamed broccoli for the steamed mixed vegetables.

NUTRITIONAL ANALYSIS (per serving):
Total carbohydrates: 60 g / Protein: 50 g / Fat: 7 g / Dietary fiber: 12 g / Calories: 490

Easy Rider Plate

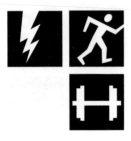

THIS SUPERCHARGED PLATE IS SO EASY AND SO GOOD, you'll turn to it time and again. No guilt when you combine these good-for-you foods. You can make this with brown rice if you prefer, or substitute steamed spinach or broccoli for the pasta.

SERVES 1

2 ounces whole wheat **FETTUCCINE** or **SPAGHETTI**

One 6-ounce can water-packed **ALBACORE TUNA**, drained

½ cup plus 2 tablespoons **THE PUMP'S HOMEMADE TOMATO SAUCE**, page 110

Preheat the oven to 375°F.

Cook the pasta in a saucepan of rapidly boiling water for about 8 minutes or until al dente. Drain and transfer to a small baking dish (a pie plate works well).

In a bowl, flake the tuna with a fork. Add the tomato sauce and mix well.

Spoon the tuna mixture over the pasta and bake for 10 to 12 minutes or until hot and bubbly. Serve immediately.

NUTRITIONAL ANALYSIS (per serving):
Total carbohydrates: 49 g / Protein: 48 g / Fat: 10 g / Dietary fiber: 4 g / Calories: 490

Flying High Plate

THIS PLATE IS TERRIFIC FOR ANYONE WHO IS BULKING UP and working out hard at the gym. While it's not really for dieters, you can try it if you substitute steamed veggies for the pasta. The cheese makes all the difference here and satisfies all cravings for something hot and oozingly delicious.

SERVES 1

2 ounces whole wheat **FETTUCCINE** or **SPAGHETTI**

1 serving **GRILLED LEMON CHICKEN**, sliced, page 91

½ cup plus 2 tablespoons **THE PUMP'S HOMEMADE TOMATO SAUCE**, page 110

4 ounces nonfat **MOZZARELLA,** shredded

Preheat the oven to 375°F.

Cook the pasta in a saucepan of rapidly boiling water for about 8 minutes or until al dente. Drain and transfer to a small baking dish (a pie plate works well).

Top the pasta with the chicken and tomato sauce. Sprinkle the cheese evenly over the sauce. Bake for 8 to 10 minutes or until hot and bubbly. Serve immediately.

NUTRITIONAL ANALYSIS (per serving):
Total carbohydrates: 54 g / Protein: 64 g / Fat: 7 g / Dietary fiber: 7 g / Calories: 540

Gigante Plate

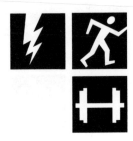

FOR SOMETHING A LITTLE DIFFERENT, try this unusual combination of brown rice and egg whites. Lots of protein equals lots of energy! Eat it for breakfast or lunch, and if you like a little spice in life, add the hot pepper sauce.

SERVES 1

½ cup cooked **BROWN RICE**, page 139
5 large **EGG WHITES**, whisked

¼ cup hot **VEGETARIAN CHILI**, page 99
HOT PEPPER SAUCE, optional

Preheat the oven to 375°F.

Spread the rice in a small baking dish (a pie plate works well). With the back of a soupspoon, make an indentation in the middle of the rice. Pour the egg whites into the indentation and bake for 8 to 10 minutes or until the eggs are set.

Pour the chili over the eggs and rice and serve immediately with hot sauce, if desired.

NUTRITIONAL ANALYSIS (per serving):
Total carbohydrates: 29 g / Protein: 22 g / Fat: 1.5 g / Dietary fiber: 3 g / Calories: 220

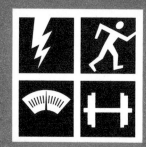

16.
The Pump Energy Two-Week Meal Plans

The Pump Slim-Down Plan

HERE IS A FAST WAY TO JUMP-START THE NEW YOU. If you combine this 14-day diet with 40 minutes of moderate exercise every day, you will lose 12 to 14 pounds and feel great in the process. This diet gives your body the food that it needs to be truly alive—to help you focus, increase your energy, and allow you to work and play with enthusiasm. The better the food you eat, the more efficient your body will be, and the more fat your body will burn.

Drink a big glass of water with every meal and snack. We recommend 14 to 16 ounces, but if that is too much for you at one time, drink at least 8 ounces. Water helps your body burn fat.

Begin each day with a piece of fruit. Fruit has a clean and natural taste, and gets us off to the right start every morning.

It's equally important to take a multivitamin pill daily. Check with your doctor or nutritionist before setting up a plan of vitamins and other supplements.

Here are some tips to make this diet work.

- Every evening, write down what you plan to eat the next day. Planning helps you avoid the wrong foods.
- Keep a running shopping list and shop for food in advance. Cheating is easy when you don't have the right foods on hand.
- Keep healthful snacks in your refrigerator at home and, if possible, at work. These include sliced cucumbers sprinkled with a little sea salt, raw cauliflower florets, celery sticks, washed and ready romaine lettuce hearts, apples, oranges, grapefruit, and pears.
- In the car or in your bag, keep small plastic bags of almonds, macadamia nuts, raisins, and figs (or make your own nut and fruit mix). Pack rice cakes, protein bars, and bottles of water, too.
- Enjoy herbal tea as a great way to relax.

Finally, we urge you to love yourself more than you love junk food! Don't let bad food take away your dreams.

Day 1

WHEN YOU WAKE UP

1 apple

BREAKFAST

The Pump's Spinach and Tomato Omelet, page 194

1 cup tea or coffee (regular or decaffeinated), optional. Add a teaspoon or so of 2% milk and a drop of half-and-half, if you want, or add a little soy milk or rice milk.

SNACK

10 to 12 almonds

1/2 ounce dried papaya

LUNCH

Classic Green Salad, page 42

Grilled Lemon Chicken, page 91

SNACK

1 cup nonfat frozen yogurt or one 6- to 8-ounce container low-fat yogurt

DINNER

Classic Green Salad, page 42

Halibut with Fresh Ginger, page 68

Steamed Spinach, page 138

DESSERT

1 cup raspberries

BEFORE BED

1 cup unsweetened herbal tea (your choice)

Day 2

WHEN YOU WAKE UP

1 orange

BREAKFAST

One 1.3-ounce serving packet of plain oatmeal with a scoop of protein powder (1/4 to 1/3 cup) of choice. Moisten the oatmeal with skim milk, 2% milk, soy milk, or rice milk, if desired.

6 sliced strawberries

1 cup tea or coffee (regular or decaffeinated), optional. Add a teaspoon or so of 2% milk and a drop of half-and-half, if you want, or add a little soy milk or rice milk.

SNACK

Half a 2-ounce protein bar (your favorite brand)

LUNCH

Sliced Turkey Breast, page 92

Pump Salad, page 38

1 cup Lentil Soup, page 29

SNACK

Half a 2-ounce protein bar (your favorite brand)

DINNER

Romaine Dill Salad, page 43

Strip Steak with Mushrooms and Peppers, page 76

Steamed Green and White Vegetables, page 124

DESSERT

1/2 cup natural, unsweetened applesauce

BEFORE BED

1 cup unsweetened herbal tea (your choice)

Day 3

WHEN YOU WAKE UP

1 Pear

BREAKFAST

Half a cantaloupe with 1/2 cup low-fat cottage cheese mixed with a scoop of protein powder (1/4 to 1/3 cup) of choice

1 cup tea or coffee (regular or decaffeinated), optional. Add a teaspoon or so of 2% milk and a drop of half-and-half, if you want, or add a little soy milk or rice milk.

SNACK

10 to 12 macadamia nuts

20 white seedless grapes

LUNCH

Tuna Salad Sandwich with Hummus, page 34

1 apple

SNACK

Blueberry-Apple Protein Shake, page 161

DINNER

Green Cabbage Salad, page 49

Lean Body Supercharged Plate, page 219

DESSERT

Baked Pineapple with Strawberry Sauce, page 178

BEFORE BED

1 cup unsweetened herbal tea (your choice)

Day 4

WHEN YOU WAKE UP

1/2 grapefruit

BREAKFAST

Rice Cake Cereal Snack, page 210

1 cup tea or coffee (regular or decaffeinated), optional. Add a teaspoon or so of 2% milk and a drop of half-and-half, if you want, or add a little soy milk or rice milk.

SNACK

Papaya Protein Shake, page 153

LUNCH

Baked Tofu, page 98

Pump Salad, page 38

SNACK

4 dried figs

DINNER

Three-Bean Salad, page 45

Quinoa with Vegetables, page 100

DESSERT

The Pump's Fruit Salad, page 186

BEFORE BED

1 cup unsweetened herbal tea (your choice)

Day 5

WHEN YOU WAKE UP

1 orange

BREAKFAST

Banana-Strawberry Soy Protein Shake, page 160

1 slice whole wheat toast with a teaspoon of
100% fruit spread

1 cup tea or coffee (regular or decaffeinated),
optional. Add a teaspoon or so of 2% milk
and a drop of half-and-half, if you want, or
add a little soy milk or rice milk.

SNACK

1 apple

LUNCH

Grilled Lemon Chicken Sandwich, page 31

Vegetarian Chili, page 99

SNACK

1 apple

DINNER

Cucumber and Watercress Salad, page 48

Baked Salmon with Tomato Salsa, page 69

DESSERT

Baked Pineapple with Strawberry Sauce,
page 178. Substitute a pear for the
pineapple, see recipe note.

BEFORE BED

1 cup unsweetened herbal tea (your choice)

Day 6

WHEN YOU WAKE UP

1 pear

BREAKFAST

Egg Delight Sandwich, page 200

1 cup tea or coffee (regular or decaffeinated),
optional. Add a teaspoon or so of 2% milk
and a drop of half-and-half, if you want, or
add a little soy milk or rice milk.

SNACK

Frozen Yogurt with Protein, page 212

LUNCH

Lean and Mean Supercharged Plate, page 217
(can be topped with Lentil Soup, page 29)

SNACK

25 red seedless grapes

DINNER

Tomato-Basil Salad, page 39

Herbed Lamb Chops, page 84

Baked Zucchini, page 127

DESSERT

Blueberry-Apple Protein Shake, page 161

BEFORE BED

1 cup unsweetened herbal tea (your choice)

Day 7

Day 8

I have a client from Blacksburg, Virginia, who runs marathons. He comes to New York every other month and when he's here he forgoes the Four Seasons and Gramercy Tavern to order from Pump. His dream is to have a Pump near him in Blacksburg.
—STU SELTZER

Day 7

WHEN YOU WAKE UP
1 apple

BREAKFAST
Rice Cakes with Fruity Cottage Cheese, page 209
1 cup tea or coffee (regular or decaffeinated), optional. Add a teaspoon or so of 2% milk and a drop of half-and-half, if you want, or add a little soy milk or rice milk.

SNACK
1 cup of Lentil Soup, page 29 (add 1/4 cup brown rice, page 139, to the soup, if you want)

LUNCH
Our Favorite Salad, page 44
Grilled Lemon Chicken, page 91

SNACK
Creativity Juice, page 162

DINNER
Steak Pizzaiola, page 79
1 1/2 cups of steamed broccoli florets

DESSERT
1 cup fresh blueberries

BEFORE BED
1 cup unsweetened herbal tea (your choice)

Day 8

WHEN YOU WAKE UP
1/2 grapefruit

BREAKFAST
One 1.3-ounce packet of plain oatmeal with a scoop of protein powder (1/4 to 1/3 cup) of choice. Moisten the oatmeal with skim milk, 2% milk, soy milk, or rice milk, if desired.
6 sliced strawberries
1 cup tea or coffee (regular or decaffeinated), optional. Add a teaspoon or so of 2% milk and a drop of half-and-half, if you want, or add a little soy milk or rice milk.

SNACK
4 figs

LUNCH
Tuna Salad (from Tuna Salad Sandwich with Hummus, page 34)
1/4 cup brown rice, page 139

SNACK
10 to 12 almonds
1 1/2 ounce piece of dried papaya

DINNER
Classic Green Salad, page 42
Fillet of Flounder with Pesto, page 72
Warm Asparagus and Snow Pea Salad, page 128

DESSERT
1/2 cup natural unsweetened applesauce

BEFORE BED
1 cup unsweetened herbal tea (your choice)

Day 9

WHEN YOU WAKE UP

1 apple

BREAKFAST

Turbo Chicken Omelet, page 193

1 cup tea or coffee (regular or decaffeinated), optional. Add a teaspoon or so of 2% milk and a drop of half-and-half, if you want, or add a little soy milk or rice milk.

SNACK

Half a 2-ounce protein bar (your favorite brand)

LUNCH

Nature Burger, page 117

Pump Salad, page 38

Vegetarian Chili, page 99

SNACK

Half a 2-ounce protein bar
   (your favorite brand)

DINNER

Romaine Dill Salad, page 43

Baked Salmon with Tomato Salsa, page 69

Baked Zucchini, page 127

BEFORE BED

1 cup unsweetened herbal tea (your choice)

Day 10

WHEN YOU WAKE UP

1 pear

BREAKFAST

Chocolate Whey Protein Shake, page 158

1 slice whole wheat toast with a teaspoon of
   100% fruit spread

1 cup tea or coffee (regular or decaffeinated), optional. Add a teaspoon or so of 2% milk and a drop of half-and-half, if you want, or add a little soy milk or rice milk.

SNACK

Carrot–Sweet Potato Soup, page 28

LUNCH

Greek Salad, page 51

SNACK

½ cup nonfat cottage cheese

DINNER

Pump Salad, page 38

The Lean Body Supercharged Plate, page 219

EVENING SNACK

2 cups plain, unbuttered popcorn

BEFORE BED

1 cup unsweetened herbal tea (your choice)

Day 11 Day 12

Day 11

WHEN YOU WAKE UP

1 orange

BREAKFAST

Half a cantaloupe with ½ cup low-fat cottage
cheese. You can mix a scoop (¼ to ⅓ cup)
of soy or whey protein into the cottage
cheese.

1 cup tea or coffee (regular or decaffeinated),
optional. Add a teaspoon or so of 2% milk
and a drop of half-and-half, if you want, or
add a little soy milk or rice milk.

SNACK

Thick Coffee Shake, page 151

LUNCH

Champion Supercharged Plate, page 218

SNACK

1 cup The Pump Chicken Soup, page 24

DINNER

Black Bean and Corn Salad, page 60
Baked Tofu, page 98

DESSERT

Baked Pineapple with Strawberry Sauce,
page 178

Day 12

WHEN YOU WAKE UP

½ grapefruit

BREAKFAST

The Pump's Pepper and Mushroom Omelet,
page 196

1 cup tea or coffee (regular or decaffeinated),
optional. Add a teaspoon or so of 2% milk
and a drop of half-and-half, if you want, or
add a little soy milk or rice milk.

SNACK

12 macadamia nuts
20 white seedless grapes

LUNCH

The New York Sandwich, page 33

SNACK

1 cup nonfat frozen yogurt or one 6- to 8-ounce
container low-fat yogurt

DINNER

Cucumber and Watercress Salad, page 48
Steak with Thyme and Mustard, page 78

DESSERT

Apple-Strawberry Shake, page 149

BEFORE BED

1 cup unsweetened herbal tea (your choice)

Day 13

WHEN YOU WAKE UP
1 pear
BREAKFAST
Rice Cakes with Banana, page 208
1 cup tea or coffee (regular or decaffeinated),
  optional. Add a teaspoon or so of 2% milk
  and a drop of half-and-half, if you want, or
  add a little soy milk or rice milk.
SNACK
The Pump Energy Shake, page 159
LUNCH
Super-Balanced Baked Turkey Omelet, page 198
SNACK
1 cup of Vegetarian Chili, page 99 (add ¼ cup
  brown rice, page 139, to the chili if you want)
DINNER
Green Leaf Lettuce Salad with Cilantro, page 53
Ginger-Tofu Stir-Fry, page 105
DESSERT
Blueberries and Strawberries with Yogurt,
  page 211
BEFORE BED
1 cup unsweetened herbal tea (your choice)

Day 14

WHEN YOU WAKE UP
1 apple
BREAKFAST
Egg, Tofu, and Tomato Sandwich, page 00
1 cup tea or coffee (regular or decaffeinated),
  optional. Add a teaspoon or so of 2% milk
  and a drop of half-and-half, if you want, or
  add a little soy milk or rice milk.
SNACK
Chocolate Peanut Butter Protein Pudding,
  page 180
LUNCH
Pump Salad, page 38
Dynamite Pita Sandwich, page 30
SNACK
Carrot-Apple-Celery Juice, page 164
DINNER
Green Cabbage Salad, page 49
Baked Chicken with Sun-Dried Tomatoes and
  Capers, page 89
1½ cups of steamed spinach, page 138
DESSERT
Baked Pineapple with Strawberry Sauce, page
  178. Substitute a pear for the pineapple,
  see recipe note.
BEFORE BED
1 cup unsweetened herbal tea (your choice)

The Pump Muscle Plan

WHEN YOU WORK OUT A LOT AND CONCENTRATE ON BUILDING MUSCLE, you should do everything else right, too. This means getting plenty of sleep, relaxation, fresh air, sunshine, and—of course—the right food.

This is where we can help. We've put together two weeks of a diet designed for anyone who wants to build muscle without putting on excess fat. The secret to our diet is that it has no gimmicks—just good, real food. There are lots of vegetables and good-for-you complex carbohydrates such as brown rice, sweet potatoes, quinoa, and oatmeal. We also recommend fresh fruit. It contains more natural sugars than do vegetables, but when you are hitting the gym, you can and should eat fruit. All these foods are important to help you digest and process the kind of high-protein diet that provides optimal energy.

For protein, we suggest lean meat, poultry, and fish. We also rely on legumes, egg whites, and handfuls of beneficial nuts. As crucial as protein is, so is fat. Not too much, of course, but healthful fats such as almond butter, flaxseed oil, and avocados keep your body working like clockwork.

Drinking shakes spiked with protein powder and protein and carbohydrate powder adds to your success. We make suggestions here for some of our favorite shakes, but look through the recipes in Chapter 10 and select those that appeal to you. We recommend adding protein powders to shakes that don't already have them if you are trying to build muscle. Usually a scoop does the trick, and depending on the brand of powder, the scoop will measure from 1/4 to 1/3 cup.

When you follow our diet plan or when you eat any of the dishes in this book, always drink a big glass of water with your meal. We recommend 14 to 16 ounces with every meal and snack, but if that is too much for you at one time, drink at least an 8-ounce glass and sip water between meals.

Building muscle and developing a buff body takes work. Approach it like a job. Don't shirk any aspect of the process and you'll be on your way to optimal health and well-being the Pump way.

Day 1

WHEN YOU WAKE UP
Creamy Orange-Banana Meal-Substitute Shake, page 148

BREAKFAST
Turbo Chicken Omelet, page 193
Simply Cooked Sweet Potatoes, page 135
2 slices whole wheat toast, each with 1 tablespoon almond butter
1 cup tea or coffee (regular or decaffeinated), optional. Add a teaspoon or so of 2% milk and a drop of half-and-half, if you want, or add a little soy milk or rice milk.

SNACK
Quick Tuna Fix (with a rice cake), page 206

LUNCH
Diesel Supercharged Plate, page 221
Steamed Green and White Vegetables, page 124

SNACK
Sweet Potato and Banana Pie, page 184
Chocolate Whey Protein Shake, page 158

DINNER
The Rock Supercharged Plate, page 223

LATE NIGHT SNACK
Frozen Yogurt with Protein, page 212

Day 2

WHEN YOU WAKE UP
Thick Coffee Shake, page 151, made with one about 2 1/2-ounce package protein and carbohydrate powder

BREAKFAST
Two 1.3-ounce serving packets of plain oatmeal with 2 scoops protein powder (1/4 to 1/3 cup) of choice and 2 tablespoons flaxseed oil. Moisten the oatmeal with skim milk, 2% milk, soy milk, or rice milk, if desired.
6 sliced strawberries
1 cup tea or coffee (regular or decaffeinated), optional. Add a teaspoon or so of 2% milk and a drop of half-and-half, if you want, or add a little soy milk or rice milk.

SNACK
Grilled Lemon Chicken, page 91
Pumped-Up Hummus, page 16

LUNCH
2 Rookie Steak Burgers, page 119

SNACK
Pump Apple Pie, page 182
Strawberry-Banana Shake, page 144, made with whey protein powder

DINNER
Three-Bean Salad, page 45
Baked Salmon with Cauliflower and Lemon Sauce, page 71

RUN OVER, DAY 2
EVENING SNACK
5 large egg whites, scrambled
2 slices whole wheat toast, each with 1 tablespoon almond butter and 1 teaspoon 100% fruit spread

When I visit New York to do a concert or appearance I always enjoy the Pump's mouthwatering food to get me ready. I know that my blood sugar will remain at a normal level . . . the body gets plenty of vital protein, vitamins, and minerals, and I have energy to burn. Thank you, Steve and Elena, for creating the Pump. It is an inspiration for people of all ages.
—JON MIKL THOR,
Mr. Canada, Mr. USA,
Actor/Musician

Day 3

WHEN YOU WAKE UP

Carrot-Orange Shake, page 146, made with
   whey protein

BREAKFAST

3 Pump's Protein Pancakes, page 202, with
   2 tablespoons almond butter; 2 tablespoons
   pure maple syrup or 100% fruit spread are
   optional.

1 cup tea or coffee (regular or decaffeinated),
   optional. Add a teaspoon or so of 2% milk
   and a drop of half-and-half, if you want, or
   add a little soy milk or rice milk.

SNACK

Steak-and-Egg Sandwich, page 199

LUNCH

Muscle Power Supercharged Plate, page 216

1 apple

SNACK

2-ounce protein bar

DINNER

Warm Asparagus and Snow Pea Salad, page 128

Flank Steak with Green Peppers and Onion
   Flakes, page 81

DESSERT

Baked Pineapple with Strawberry Sauce, page
   178

Blueberry-Apple Protein Shake, page 161,
   made with whey protein

Day 4

WHEN YOU WAKE UP

Tropical Island Shake, page 155, made with
   whey protein

BREAKFAST

The Pump's Spinach and Tomato Omelet,
   page 194

1 cup brown rice, page 139

4 ounces Sliced Turkey Breast, page 92

1 cup tea or coffee (regular or decaffeinated),
   optional. Add a teaspoon or so of 2% milk
   and a drop of half-and-half, if you want, or
   add a little soy milk or rice milk.

SNACK

2-ounce protein bar

30 seedless white grapes

LUNCH

Champion Supercharged Plate, page 218

Vegetarian Chili, page 99

SNACK

Sweet Potato and Banana Pie, page 184

Thick Coffee Shake, page 151, made with
   whey protein powder

DINNER

Romaine Dill Salad, page 43

Baked Chicken Breast with Lemongrass, Lime,
   and Orange, page 90

EVENING SNACK

Blueberries and strawberries with whole plain
   yogurt. Mix 1 scoop of protein powder ($1/4$ to
   $1/3$ cup) into the yogurt.

Day 5

WHEN YOU WAKE UP
Peaches-and-Cream Shake, page 152, made
with whey protein powder

BREAKFAST
Two 1.3-ounce serving packets of plain oatmeal
with 2 scoops protein powder (1/4 to 1/3 cup)
of choice and 2 tablespoons flaxseed oil.
Moisten the oatmeal with skim milk, 2%
milk, soy milk, or rice milk, if desired.
6 sliced strawberries
1 cup tea or coffee (regular or decaffeinated),
optional. Add a teaspoon or so of 2% milk
and a drop of half-and-half, if you want, or
add a little soy milk or rice milk.

SNACK
1 cup brown rice, page 139
Grilled Lemon Chicken, page 91
Guacamole the Pump Way, page 14

LUNCH
Gigante Supercharged Plate, page 226

SNACK
Summer Shake, page 150, made with
1 package (about 2 1/2 ounces) protein
and carbohydrate powder

DINNER
Grilled Sirloin with Portobello Mushrooms and
Onions, page 80
Eggplant Carpaccio, page 133
Simply Cooked Sweet Potatoes, page 135

EVENING SNACK
The Pump's Fruit Salad, page 186
1 cup cottage cheese

Day 6

WHEN YOU WAKE UP
Mixed Fruit Shake, page 157, made with
1 package (about 2 1/2 ounces) protein and
carbohydrate powder

BREAKFAST
Super-Balanced Baked Turkey Omelet, page 198
1 slice whole wheat toast with 1 tablespoon of
almond butter
1 cup tea or coffee (regular or decaffeinated),
optional. Add a teaspoon or so of 2% milk
and a drop of half-and-half, if you want, or
add a little soy milk or rice milk.

SNACK
Dynamite Pita Sandwich, page 30

LUNCH
Dionysus Supercharged Plate, page 222

SNACK
Tuna Salad (from Tuna Salad with Hummus
Sandwich), page 34

DINNER
Red Kidney Bean Salad with Fresh Tomatoes,
page 59
Chicken with Spinach and Ricotta, page 86

EVENING SNACK
Baked Pineapple with Strawberry Sauce, page
178. Substitute a pear for the pineapple, see
recipe note.

Over the last four months
I have returned to the gym
and now of the fifteen
meals I normally eat, twelve
are from the Pump (I take
home two dinners per
week). I have already lost
22 pounds of the 50 plus
I intend to lose. In this rela-
tively short period of time,
I have lost fat and added
quite a bit of muscle. I love
the taste and variety of the
food. My energy levels are
way up, I sleep better, and
I am not as tired as I used
to be. Your food tastes great
and my life is much better.
—Ric DiBartolo

Day 7

WHEN YOU WAKE UP
Papaya Protein Shake, page 153

BREAKFAST
Turbo Chicken Omelet, page 193
1 Pump's Protein Pancake, page 202, with
    1 tablespoon almond butter and 1 teaspoon
    100% fruit spread

SNACK
1 cup of Carrot–Sweet Potato Soup, page 28
1 cup of Pump Chicken Soup, page 24

LUNCH
2 Chicken and Spinach Sandwiches, page 32

SNACK
One 2-ounce protein bar
1 cup blueberries

DINNER
Pump Salad, page 38
Halibut with Fresh Ginger, page 68
1 cup brown rice, page 139

EVENING SNACK
½ cantaloupe with 1 cup cottage cheese

Day 8

WHEN YOU WAKE UP
Creamy Orange-Banana Meal-Substitute Shake,
    page 148

BREAKFAST
Steak-and-Egg Sandwich, page 199
Simply Cooked Sweet Potatoes, page 135
1 cup tea or coffee (regular or decaffeinated),
    optional. Add a teaspoon or so of 2% milk
    and a drop of half-and-half, if you want, or
    add a little soy milk or rice milk.

SNACK
Chunky Oil-Free Avocado Salsa, page 15
The Pump's Baked Falafel, page 17

LUNCH
The Rock Supercharged Plate, page 223
1 apple

SNACK
Pizza-Style Turkey Burger, page 120
Creativity Juice, page 162

DINNER
Asian Peanut Stir-Fry, page 104
Pan-Seared Scallops with Stewed Tomatoes and
    Parsnips, page 65

EVENING SNACK
Pump Apple Pie, page 182
15 almonds

Day 9

WHEN YOU WAKE UP

Apple-Strawberry Shake, page 149, made with
whey protein powder

BREAKFAST

3 Pump's Protein Pancakes, page 202, with 2
tablespoons almond butter and 3
tablespoons pure maple syrup or 100% fruit
spread

1/2 cup cottage cheese

5 sliced strawberries

1 cup tea or coffee (regular or decaffeinated),
optional. Add a teaspoon or so of 2% milk
and a drop of half-and-half, if you want, or
add a little soy milk or rice milk.

SNACK

2-ounce protein bar (your favorite brand)

30 red seedless grapes

LUNCH

Easy Rider Supercharged Plate, page 224

Simply Cooked Sweet Potatoes, page 135

SNACK

Rookie Steak Burger, page 119

DINNER

Asparagus Salad, page 55

Steak Pizzaiola, page 79

1/2 cup brown rice, page 139

EVENING SNACK

2 slices whole wheat toast, each with 1 tablespoon almond butter and 1 teaspoon 100%
fruit spread

5 large scrambled egg whites

Day 10

WHEN YOU WAKE UP

Carrot-Orange Shake, page 146, made with
1 package (about 2 1/2 ounces) protein and
carbohydrate powder

BREAKFAST

The Pump's Broccoli and Mozzarella Omelet,
page 195

Simply Cooked Sweet Potatoes, page 135

1 cup tea or coffee (regular or decaffeinated),
optional. Add a teaspoon or so of 2% milk
and a drop of half-and-half, if you want, or
add a little soy milk or rice milk.

SNACK

Tuna Salad with Hummus Sandwich, page 34

LUNCH

Diesel Supercharged Plate, page 221

1 cup steamed spinach, page 138

SNACK

The Pump Chicken Soup, page 24

5 large scrambled egg whites

DINNER

French Bean and Tomato Salad, page 61

Strip Steak with Mushrooms and Peppers,
page 76

1/2 cup brown rice, page 139

EVENING SNACK

Frozen Yogurt with Protein, page 212

1 cup raspberries

Day 11

WHEN YOU WAKE UP

Papaya Protein Shake, page 153

BREAKFAST

Two 1.3-ounce serving packets of plain oatmeal with 2 scoops protein powder of choice (1/4 to 1/3 cup) and 2 tablespoons flaxseed oil. Moisten the oatmeal with skim milk, 2% milk, soy milk, or rice milk, if desired.

1 cup tea or coffee (regular or decaffeinated), optional. Add a teaspoon or so of 2% milk and a drop of half-and-half, if you want, or add a little soy milk or rice milk.

SNACK

Egg Delight Sandwich, page 200

LUNCH

Flying High Supercharged Plate, page 225

SNACK

2-ounce protein bar (your choice)

30 white seedless grapes

DINNER

Romaine Dill Salad, page 43

Baked Salmon with Tomato Salsa, page 69

Quinoa with Dill, page 131

DESSERT

Pump Apple Pie, page 182

10 sliced strawberries

Day 12

WHEN YOU WAKE UP

Mixed Fruit Shake, page 157, made with 1 package (about 2 1/2 ounces) protein and carbohydrate powder

BREAKFAST

The Pump's Pepper and Mushroom Omelet, page 196

Simply Cooked Sweet Potatoes, page 135

1 slice whole wheat toast with 1 tablespoon almond butter and 1 teaspoon 100% fruit spread

1 cup tea or coffee (regular or decaffeinated), optional. Add a teaspoon or so of 2% milk and a drop of half-and-half, if you want, or add a little soy milk or rice milk.

SNACK

Chicken and Spinach Sandwich, page 32

LUNCH

Three-Bean Salad, page 45

Grilled Lemon Chicken, page 91

SNACK

Sweet Potato and Banana Pie, page 184

Thick Coffee Shake, page 151, made with whey protein powder

DINNER

Chickpea Stew with Basil, page 101

Chopped Sirloin with Basil and Steamed String Beans, page 82

DESSERT

Baked Pineapple with Strawberry Sauce, page 178

1/2 cup cottage cheese

Day 13

WHEN YOU WAKE UP
Strawberry-Banana Shake, page 144, made
   with whey protein powder

BREAKFAST
Two 1.3-ounce serving packets of plain oatmeal
   with 2 scoops protein powder of choice (1/4
   to 1/3 cup) and 2 tablespoons flaxseed oil.
   Moisten the oatmeal with skim milk, 2%
   milk, soy milk, or rice milk, if desired.
1 cup tea or coffee (regular or decaffeinated),
   optional. Add a teaspoon or so of 2% milk
   and a drop of half-and-half, if you want, or
   add a little soy milk or rice milk.

SNACK
Tuna Salad with Hummus Sandwich, page 34

LUNCH
2 Chicken-Spinach Pizzas, page 113

SNACK
1 cup Vegetarian Chili, page 99 (add 1/4 cup
   brown rice, page 139, to the chili if you want)
5 large scrambled egg whites

DINNER
Green Leaf Lettuce Salad with Cilantro, page 53
Marinated Rosemary-Garlic Chicken, page 88

DESSERT
2-ounce protein bar (your choice)
30 seedless red grapes

Day 14

WHEN YOU WAKE UP
Peaches-and-Cream Shake, page 152, made
   with whey protein powder

BREAKFAST
3 Pump's Protein Pancakes, page 202, with
   2 tablespoons almond butter and 3 tablespoons pure maple syrup or 100% fruit
   spread
1 cup tea or coffee (regular or decaffeinated),
   optional. Add a teaspoon or so of 2% milk
   and a drop of half-and-half, if you want, or
   add a little soy milk or rice milk.

SNACK
1 cup brown rice, page 139
Sliced Turkey Breast, page 92
Guacamole the Pump Way, page 14

LUNCH
2 Steak-and-Onion Pizzas, page 112

SNACK
Sweet Potato and Banana Pie, page 184
1/2 cup cottage cheese

DINNER
Our Favorite Salad, page 44
Herbed Lamb Chops, page 84
Crispy Sliced Potatoes, page 132

EVENING SNACK
10 sliced strawberries
10 almonds

Index

Appetizers, 13–21
  Baked Cauliflower, 18
  Cheese-Topped Baked
      Portobello Mushrooms, 21
  Chunky Oil-Free Avocado
      Salsa, 15
  Guacamole the Pump Way, 14
  Herbed Shallot-Stuffed
      Portobello Mushrooms, 19
  Pumped-Up Hummus, 16
  The Pump's Baked Falafel, 17
Apple:
  -Blueberry Protein Shake, 161
  -Carrot-Celery Juice, 164
  Get-Up-and-Go Juice, 163
  Pie, Pump, 182–83
  Stewed Fruit with Orange
      Juice and Yogurt, 179
  -Strawberry Shake, 149
Artichoke Salad, Fresh, 56–57
Asian Peanut Stir-Fry, 104
Asparagus:
  Salad, 55
  and Snow Pea Salad, Warm,
      128
Avocado:
  Black Bean and Corn Salad,
      60
  Chunky Oil-Free Salsa, 15
  Guacamole the Pump Way, 14

Our Favorite Salad, 44

Baked Cauliflower Appetizer, 18
Baked Chicken Breast with
    Lemongrass, 90
Baked Chicken Breast with
    Stewed Peaches, 85
Baked Chicken with Sun-Dried
    Tomatoes, 89
Baked Pineapple with Strawberry
    Sauce, 178
Baked Salmon with Cauliflower
    and Lemon Sauce, 71
Baked Salmon with Tomato
    Salsa, 69
Baked Tofu, 98
Baked Zucchini, 127
Ball games, tips for, 9
Banana:
  Frozen, Shake, 145
  how to freeze, 148
  –Peanut Butter Chocolate
      Shake, 154
  Rice Cakes with, 208
  Stewed Fruit with Orange
      Juice and Yogurt, 179
  -Strawberry Shake, 144
  -Strawberry Soy Protein
      Shake, 160
  and Sweet Potato Pie, 184–85

Basil:
  Chickpea Stew with, 101
  Chopped Sirloin with String
      Beans and, 82
  Fillet of Flounder with Pesto, 72
  Tomato Salad with Thyme
      Vinaigrette, 39
Beans:
  Black, and Corn Salad, 60
  dried, how to cook, 107
  French, and Tomato Salad, 61
  Kidney, and Butternut Squash
      Stew, 102
  Red, Salad Finale with Cilantro
      and, 54
  Red Kidney, Salad with Fresh
      Tomatoes, 59
  String, Chopped Sirloin with
      Basil and, 82
  String, Salad, 58
  Tahini Dressing, 175
  Three, Salad of, 45
  Vegetarian Chili, 99
Beautiful and Delicious Chickpea
    Salad, 52
Berries:
  Summer Shake, 156
  with Yogurt, 211
  see also Strawberries
Black Bean and Corn Salad, 60

Black-Eyed Peas:
  how to cook, 106
  Red Cabbage Salad with, 50
Blueberries:
  -Apple Protein Shake, 161
  and Strawberries with Yogurt,
      211
Boneless Leg of Lamb with
    Roasted Vegetables, 83
Broccoli and Mozzarella Omelet,
    The Pump's, 195
Broiled Scallops with Paprika, 64
Brown rice:
  Champion Plate, 218
  Diesel Plate, 221
  Gigante Plate, 226
  how to cook, 139
  Muscle Power Plate, 216
  Nature Burger, 117
  with Peas and Carrots, 136
  The Rock Plate, 223
Buffets, party tips, 9
Burgers, 109
  Chopped Sirloin with Basil and
      String Beans, 82
  Nature, 117
  Pizza-Style Turkey, 120
  Rookie Steak, 119
  Turkey, Pizza, 114
Butternut Squash:

and Kidney Bean Stew, 102
Roasted Cinnamon, 125
Soup, 27

Cabbage:
Green, Salad, 49
Red, Salad with Black-Eyed
Peas, 50
Salad Finale with Cilantro and
Red Beans, 54
Capers, Shrimp with, 67
Carpaccio, Eggplant, 133
Carrots:
-Apple-Celery Juice, 164
Brown Rice with Peas and, 136
Dill-and-Chive Snow Peas
and, 126
Get-Up-and-Go Juice, 163
-Ginger Dressing, 174
-Orange Shake, 146
–Sweet Potato Soup, 28
Cauliflower:
Baked Appetizer, 18
Baked Salmon with Lemon
Sauce and, 71
Celery-Carrot-Apple Juice, 164
Champion Plate, 218
Cheese-Topped Baked Portobello
Mushrooms, 21
Chicken:
Baked, with Sun-Dried
Tomatoes, 89
Baked Breast with
Lemongrass, 90
Baked Breast with Stewed
Peaches, 85
Champion Plate, 218
Diesel Plate, 221

Dionysus Plate, 222
Dynamite Pita Sandwich, 30
Flying High Plate, 225
Grilled Lemon, 91
Grilled Lemon, Sandwich, 31
Lean and Mean Plate, 217
Lean Body Plate, 219
Marinated Garlic-Rosemary,
88
Muscle Power Plate, 216
The New York Sandwich, 33
with Spinach and Ricotta
Cheese, 86–87
-Spinach Pizza, 113
and Spinach Sandwich, 32
The Pump Soup, 24–25
Turbo Omelet, 193
Chickpeas:
Beautiful and Delicious Salad,
52
how to cook, 107
Pumped-Up Hummus, 16
The Pump's Baked Falafel, 17
Stew with Basil, 101
Chili, Vegetarian, 99
Chinese restaurants, tips for, 9
Chocolate:
Banana–Peanut Butter Shake,
154
–Peanut Butter Protein
Pudding, 180
Whey Protein Shake, 158
Chopped Sirloin with Basil and
String Beans, 82
Chunky Oil-Free Avocado Salsa, 15
Cilantro:
Green Leaf Lettuce Salad with,
53

Salad Finale with Red Beans
and, 54
Cinnamon Squash, Roasted, 125
Classic Green Salad, 42
Coffee Shake, Thick, 151
Corn and Black Bean Salad, 60
Cottage Cheese, Fruity, Rice
Cakes with, 209
Creamy Orange-Banana Meal-
Substitute Shake, 148
Creativity Juice, 162
Crispy Sliced Potatoes, 132
Cucumber:
Salad, 47
and Watercress Salad, 48
Yogurt Dressing, 170

Delicatessens, tips for, 9
Delicious Pesto Without Cheese,
168
Desserts, 177–86
Baked Pineapple with
Strawberry Sauce, 178
Chocolate–Peanut Butter
Protein Pudding, 180
Pump Apple Pie, 182–83
The Pump Pie Crust, 181
The Pump's Fruit Salad, 186
Stewed Fruit with Orange
Juice and Yogurt, 179
Sweet Potato and Banana Pie,
184–85
Diesel Plate, 221
Dill:
-and-Chive Snow Peas and
Carrots, 126
-Lemon Shrimp, 66
Quinoa with, 131

Romaine Salad, 43
Dionysus Plate, 222
Dressings and sauces, 167–75
Baked Pineapple with
Strawberry Sauce, 178
Carrot-Ginger Dressing, 174
Cucumber Yogurt Dressing,
170
Delicious Pesto Without
Cheese, 168
Honey-Mustard Dressing, 172
Mustard-Thyme Vinaigrette,
173
Oil and Vinegar Dressing with
Herbs, 171
The Pump's Homemade
Tomato Sauce, 110
Soy Salad Dressing, 169
Tahini Dressing, 175
Tomato-Onion-Red Pepper
Ragù, 94
see also specific salads
Dynamite Pita Sandwich, 30

Easy Rider Plate, 224
Eggplant Carpaccio, 133
Eggs, 189–201
cooking egg whites, 203
Delight Sandwich, 200
Elena's Spinach and Feta
Omelet, 197
Gigante Plate, 226
Mega Egg White Omelet, 190
Pizzaiola Egg White Omelet, 191
The Pump's Broccoli and
Mozzarella Omelet, 195
The Pump's Pepper and
Mushroom Omelet, 196

The Pump's Protein
  Pancakes, 202
The Pump's Spinach and
  Tomato Omelet, 194
and-Steak Sandwich, 199
Super-Balanced Baked Turkey
  Omelet, 198
Tofu, and Tomato Sandwich,
  201
Turbo Chicken Omelet, 193
Elena's Spinach and Feta
  Omelet, 197

Falafel, The Pump's Baked, 17
Fast food restaurants, tips for, 9
Favorite Salad, 44
Feta Cheese:
  Greek Salad, 51
  Spinach with, 134
  and Spinach Omelet, The
    Pump's, 197
Fillet of Flounder with Pesto, 72
Five-Vegetable Salad, 46
Flank Steak with Green Peppers
  and Onion Flakes, 81
Flounder, Fillet of, with Pesto, 72
Flying High Plate, 225
French Bean and Tomato Salad,
  61
Fresh Artichoke Salad, 56–57
Frozen Banana Shake, 145
Frozen Yogurt with Protein, 212
Fruit:
  Mixed, Shake, 157
  The Pump's Salad, 186
  Stewed, with Orange Juice
    and Yogurt, 179

Garlic:
  Roasted, Rib-Eye Steak with, 77
  -Rosemary Chicken,
    Marinated, 88
Get-Up-and-Go Juice, 163
Gigante Plate, 226
Ginger:
  -Carrot Dressing, 174
  Fresh, Halibut with, 68
  -Tofu Stir-Fry, 105
Grapefruit-Orange Juice, 165
Greek Salad, 51
Green Cabbage Salad, 49
Green Leaf Lettuce Salad with
  Cilantro, 53
Green Salad, Classic, 42
Grilled Lemon Chicken, 91
Grilled Lemon Chicken
  Sandwich, 31
Grilled Sirloin with Portobello
  Mushrooms, 80
Guacamole the Pump Way, 14

Halibut with Fresh Ginger, 68
Haricots Verts (French Beans)
  and Tomato Salad, 61
Herbed Lamb Chops, 84
Herbed Shallot-Stuffed Portobello
  Mushrooms, 19
Honey-Mustard Dressing, 172
Hot Zucchini Strips with Shallots,
  207
Hummus:
  Dynamite Pita Sandwich, 30
  The New York Sandwich, 33
  Pumped-Up, 16
  Tuna Salad Sandwich with, 34

Icons, 10

Japanese restaurants, tips for, 9
Juice extractor, 143
Juices, 141, 143, 162–66
  Carrot-Apple-Celery, 164
  Creativity, 162
  Get-Up-and-Go, 163
  Grapefruit-Orange, 165

Kidney Bean and Butternut
  Squash Stew, 102
Kitchen:
  essential foods in, 5
  tips, 6
  tools for, 5, 143

Lamb:
  Boneless Leg of, with Roasted
    Vegetables, 83
  Herbed Chops, 84
Lean and Mean Plate, 217
Lean Body Plate, 219
Lemon Chicken, Grilled, 91
  Sandwich, 31
Lemon-Dill Shrimp, 66
Lemongrass, Baked Chicken
  Breast with, 90
Lemon Sauce, Baked Salmon
  with Cauliflower and, 71
Lentil Soup, 29

Marinated Garlic-Rosemary
  Chicken, 88
Mayonnaise, Soy, Tuna Salad
  with, 40
Meat, 75–84
  Boneless Leg of Lamb with

Roasted Vegetables, 83
Chopped Sirloin with Basil and
  String Beans, 82
Flank Steak with Green
  Peppers and Onion
  Flakes, 81
Grilled Sirloin with Portobello
  Mushrooms, 80
Herbed Lamb Chops, 84
Rib-Eye Steak with Roasted
  Garlic, 77
Steak Pizzaiola, 79
Steak with Thyme and
  Mustard, 78
Strip Steak with Mushrooms
  and Peppers, 76
Mega Egg White Omelet, 190
Melon, The Pump's Fruit Salad,
  186
Mixed Fruit Shake, 157
Movies, tips for eating in, 9
Mozzarella and Broccoli Omelet,
  The Pump's, 195
Muscle Power Plate, 216
Mushrooms:
  Asian Peanut Stir-Fry, 104
  Cheese-Topped Baked
    Portobello, 21
  Cucumber and Watercress
    Salad, 48
  Grilled Sirloin with Portobello,
    80
  Herbed Shallot-Stuffed
    Portobello, 19
  Kidney Bean and Butternut
    Squash Stew, 102
  and Pepper Omelet, The
    Pump's, 196

Sautéed Sugar Snap Peas with, 130

Sliced, Sautéed Sun-Dried Tomatoes with, 137

Steak Pizzaiola, 79

Strip Steak with Peppers and, 76

Mustard:

-Honey Dressing, 172

Steak with Thyme and, 78

-Thyme Vinaigrette, 173

Nature Burger, 117

Dynamite Pita Sandwich, 30

The New York Sandwich, 33

and Tomato Pizza, 116

The New York Sandwich, 33

Oil and Vinegar Dressing with Herbs, 171

Omelets:

Elena's Spinach and Feta, 197

Mega Egg White, 190

Pizzaiola Egg White, 191

The Pump's Broccoli and Mozzarella, 195

The Pump's Pepper and Mushroom, 196

The Pump's Spinach and Tomato, 194

Super-Balanced Baked Turkey, 198

Turbo Chicken, 193

Onion-Tomato-Red Pepper Ragù, 94

Orange:

-Banana Meal-Substitute Creamy Shake, 148

-Carrot Shake, 146

-Grapefruit Juice, 165

Orange Juice, Stewed Fruit with Yogurt and, 179

Our Favorite Salad, 44

Outdoor fairs, tips for, 9

Pancakes, Protein, The Pump's, 202

Pan-Seared Scallops with Tomatoes and Parsnips, 65

Papaya Protein Shake, 153

Paprika, Broiled Scallops with, 64

Parsnips, Pan-Seared Scallops with Tomatoes and, 65

Party buffets, tips for, 9

Peaches:

-and-Cream Shake, 152

Stewed, Baked Chicken Breast with, 85

Peanut Butter:

–Banana Chocolate Shake, 154

–Chocolate Protein Pudding, 180

Peanut Stir-Fry, Asian, 104

Pears, as pineapple substitute, 178

Peas:

Black-Eyed, how to cook, 106

Black-Eyed, Red Cabbage Salad with, 50

Brown Rice with Carrots and, 136

dried, how to cook, 106

Snow, and Warm Asparagus Salad, 128

Snow, Dill-and-Chive Carrots and, 126

Sugar Snap, Sautéed with Mushrooms, 130

Peppers:

Green, Flank Steak with Onion Flakes and, 81

and Mushroom Omelet, The Pump's, 196

Red, -Tomato-Onion Ragù, 94

Strip Steak with Mushrooms and, 76

Pesto:

Delicious, Without Cheese, 168

Fillet of Flounder with, 72

Pie Crust, The Pump, 181

Pies:

Pump Apple, 182–83

Sweet Potato and Banana, 184–85

Pineapple, Baked, with Strawberry Sauce, 178

Pita:

Dynamite Sandwich, 30

Nature Burger in, 117

see also Pizza

Pizza, 109–16

Chicken-Spinach, 113

Nature Burger and Tomato, 116

The Pump's Homemade Tomato Sauce, 110

Steak-and-Onion, 112

-Style Turkey Burger, 120

Tofu, 115

Turkey Burger, 114

Whole Wheat Tomato, 111

Pizzaiola:

Egg White Omelet, 191

Steak, 79

Portobello Mushrooms:

Cheese-Topped Baked, 21

Grilled Sirloin with, 80

Herbed Shallot-Stuffed, 19

Potatoes, Crispy Sliced, 132

Poultry, 75, 85–94

Roast Turkey Breast for Slicing, 92–93

see also Chicken

Protein, Frozen Yogurt with, 212

Protein Pancakes, The Pump's, 202

Protein powder, in shakes, 142, 158

Pudding, Chocolate–Peanut Butter Protein, 180

Pump Apple Pie, 182–83

Pumped-Up Hummus, 16

Pump Energy Food restaurants, xiii

The Pump Energy Shake, 159

Pump Energy two-week meal plans, 229–45

Pump Muscle Plan, 238–45

Pump Slim-Down Plan, 230–37

Pump lifestyle, 4–10

bad carbohydrates, 10

cooking tools, 5

essential foods, 5

foods to avoid, 5, 10

the kitchen, 6

recharging and maintaining, 8

right foods, 4–5

snack foods, 8

success strategies, 7–9

techniques, 6

tips, 7

Winning Quarter, 6–7

Pump Muscle Plan, 238–45

The Pump Pie Crust, 181
Pump Salad, 38
Pump Slim-Down Plan, 230–37
The Pump's Baked Falafel, 17
The Pump's Broccoli and
    Mozzarella Omelet, 195
The Pump's Fruit Salad, 186
The Pump's Homemade Tomato
    Sauce, 110
The Pump's Pepper and
    Mushroom Omelet, 196
The Pump's Protein Pancakes,
    202
Pump's Spinach and Tomato
    Omelet, The 194

Quick Tuna Fix, 206
Quinoa:
    with Dill, 131
    with Vegetables, 100

Ragù, Tomato-Onion-Red
    Pepper, 94
Red Beans, Salad Finale with
    Cilantro and, 54
Red Cabbage Salad with Black-
    Eyed Peas, 50
Red Kidney Bean Salad with
    Fresh Tomatoes, 59
Restaurants, tips for, 9
Rib-Eye Steak with Roasted
    Garlic, 77
Rice Cakes:
    with Banana, 208
    Cereal Snack, 210
    with Fruity Cottage Cheese, 209
Ricotta Cheese, Chicken with
    Spinach and, 86–87

Roast Turkey Breast for Slicing,
    92–93
Roasted Cinnamon Squash, 125
The Rock Plate, 223
Romaine Dill Salad, 43
Rookie Steak Burger, 119
Rosemary-Garlic Chicken,
    Marinated, 88

Salads, 37–61
    Asparagus, 55
    Beautiful and Delicious
        Chickpea, 52
    Black Bean and Corn, 60
    Classic Green, 42
    Cucumber, 47
    Cucumber and Watercress, 48
    Finale with Cilantro and Red
        Beans, 54
    Five-Vegetable, 46
    French Bean and Tomato, 61
    Fresh Artichoke, 56–57
    Greek, 51
    Green Cabbage, 49
    Green Leaf Lettuce with
        Cilantro, 53
    Our Favorite, 44
    Pump, 38
    The Pump's Fruit, 186
    Red Cabbage with Black-Eyed
        Peas, 50
    Red Kidney Bean with Fresh
        Tomatoes, 59
    Romaine Dill, 43
    String Bean, 58
    Three-Bean, 45
    Tomato-Basil with Thyme
        Vinaigrette, 39

Tuna Sandwich with Hummus,
    34
Tuna with Soy Mayonnaise, 40
Warm Asparagus and Snow
    Pea, 128
see also Dressings and sauces
Salmon, Baked:
    with Cauliflower and Lemon
        Sauce, 71
    with Tomato Salsa, 69
Salsas:
    Chunky Oil-Free Avocado, 15
    Tomato, Baked Salmon with,
        69
Sandwiches, 23, 30–35
    Chicken and Spinach, 32
    Dynamite Pita, 30
    Egg Delight, 200
    Egg, Tofu, and Tomato, 201
    Grilled Lemon Chicken, 31
    The New York, 33
    Steak-and-Egg, 199
    Tuna Salad with Hummus, 34
    Vegetarian Special, 35
Sauces, see Dressings and sauces
Sautéed Sliced Mushrooms with
    Sun-Dried Tomatoes, 137
Sautéed Sugar Snap Peas with
    Mushrooms, 130
Scallops:
    Broiled, with Paprika, 64
    Pan-Seared, with Tomatoes
        and Parsnips, 65
Seafood, 63–72
    Baked Salmon with Cauliflower
        and Lemon Sauce, 71
    Baked Salmon with Tomato
        Salsa, 69

Broiled Scallops with Paprika,
    64
Fillet of Flounder with Pesto, 72
Halibut with Fresh Ginger, 68
Lemon-Dill Shrimp, 66
Pan-Seared Scallops with
    Tomatoes and Parsnips, 65
Shrimp with Capers, 67
Shakes, 141–61
    Apple-Strawberry, 149
    Banana–Peanut Butter
        Chocolate, 154
    Banana-Strawberry Soy
        Protein, 160
    blender for, 143
    Blueberry-Apple Protein, 161
    Carrot-Orange, 146
    Chocolate Whey Protein, 158
    Creamy Orange-Banana Meal
        Substitute, 148
    Frozen Banana, 145
    ice cubes in, 142
    Mixed Fruit, 157
    Papaya Protein, 153
    Peaches-and-Cream, 152
    with protein, 142, 158
    The Pump Energy Shake, 159
    Strawberry, 147
    Strawberry-Banana, 144
    Summer, 150
    Summer Berry, 156
    Thick Coffee, 151
    Tropical Island, 155
Shallots:
    Hot Zucchini Strips with, 207
    -Stuffed Herbed Portobello
        Mushrooms, 19
Shrimp:

with Capers, 67
Lemon-Dill, 66
Simply Cooked Sweet Potatoes,
135
Sirloin:
Chopped, with Basil and
String Beans, 82
Grilled, with Portobello
Mushrooms, 80
Snacks, 8, 205–12
Blueberries and Strawberries
with Yogurt, 211
Frozen Yogurt with Protein,
212
Hot Zucchini Strips with
Shallots, 207
Quick Tuna Fix, 206
Rice Cake Cereal, 210
Rice Cakes with Banana, 208
Rice Cakes with Fruity Cottage
Cheese, 209
Snow Peas:
Dill-and-Chive Carrots and,
126
and Warm Asparagus Salad,
128
Soups, 23–29
Butternut Squash, 27
Carrot--Sweet Potato, 28
Lentil, 29
The Pump Chicken, 24–25
Tofu-Vegetable, 26
Soy Mayonnaise, Tuna Salad
with, 40
Soy Protein Banana-Strawberry
Shake, 160
Soy Salad Dressing, 169
Spinach:

-Chicken Pizza, 113
and Chicken Sandwich, 32
Chicken with Ricotta Cheese
with, 86–87
Creativity Juice, 162
with Feta Cheese, 134
and Feta Omelet, Elena's, 197
how to steam, 138
Lean Body Plate, 219
Muscle Power Plate, 216
and Tomato Omelet, The
Pump's, 194
Squash:
Baked Zucchini, 127
Butternut, and Kidney Bean
Stew, 102
Butternut, Soup, 27
Hot Zucchini Strips with
Shallots, 207
Roasted Cinnamon, 125
Stacks, Tomato, 129
Steak:
-and-Egg Sandwich, 199
-and-Onion Pizza, 112
Chopped Sirloin with Basil and
String Beans, 82
Dynamite Pita Sandwich, 30
Flank, with Green Peppers
and Onion Flakes, 81
Grilled Sirloin with Portobello
Mushrooms, 80
The New York Sandwich, 33
Pizzaiola, 79
Rib-Eye, with Roasted Garlic,
77
Rookie Burger, 119
Strip, with Mushrooms and
Peppers, 76

with Thyme and Mustard, 78
Steamed Green and White
Vegetables, 124
Stewed Fruit with Orange Juice
and Yogurt, 179
Stewed Peaches, Baked Chicken
Breast with, 85
Stews:
Chickpea with Basil, 101
Kidney Bean and Butternut
Squash, 102
Stir-Fry:
Asian Peanut, 104
Ginger-Tofu, 105
Strawberries:
-Apple Shake, 149
-Banana Shake, 144
-Banana Soy Protein Shake,
160
and Blueberries with Yogurt,
211
Mixed Fruit Shake, 157
The Pump's Fruit Salad, 186
Sauce, Baked Pineapple with,
178
Shake, 147
Stewed Fruit with Orange
Juice and Yogurt, 179
Summer Berry Shake, 156
String Beans:
Chopped Sirloin with Basil
and, 82
Salad, 58
Strip Steak with Mushrooms and
Peppers, 76
Sugar Snap Peas with
Mushrooms, Sautéed, 130
Summer Berry Shake, 156

Summer Shake, 150
Sun-Dried Tomatoes:
Baked Chicken with, 89
Sautéed Sliced Mushrooms
with, 137
Super-Balanced Baked Turkey
Omelet, 198
Super-charged plates, 215–26
Champion, 218
Diesel, 221
Dionysus, 222
Easy Rider, 224
Flying High, 225
Gigante, 226
Lean and Mean, 217
Lean Body, 219
Muscle Power, 216
The Rock, 223
Sweet Potatoes:
and Banana Pie, 184–85
--Carrot Soup, 28
Simply Cooked, 135

Tahini Dressing, 175
Thick Coffee Shake, 151
Three-Bean Salad, 45
Thyme:
-Mustard Vinaigrette, 173
Steak with Mustard and, 78
Vinaigrette, Tomato-Basil
Salad with, 39
Tofu:
Baked, 98
Egg, and Tomato Sandwich,
201
-Ginger Stir-Fry, 105
Pizza, 115
-Vegetable Soup, 26

Tomatoes:

-Basil Salad with Thyme
Vinaigrette, 39

Egg, and Tofu Sandwich, 201

and French Bean Salad, 61

Fresh, Red Kidney Bean Salad
with, 59

-Onion-Red Pepper Ragù, 94

Our Favorite Salad, 44

Pan-Seared Scallops with
Parsnips and, 65

Salsa, Baked Salmon with, 69

and Spinach Omelet, The
Pump's, 194

Stacks, 129

Sun-Dried, Baked Chicken
with, 89

Sun-Dried, Sautéed Sliced
Mushrooms with, 137

Whole Wheat Pizza, 111

Tomato Sauce:

and Nature Burger Pizza, 116

The Pump's Homemade, 110

Travel tips, 73

Tropical Island Shake, 155

Tuna:

Easy Rider Plate, 224

Quick Fix, 206

The Rock Plate, 223

Salad Sandwich with

Hummus, 34

Salad with Soy Mayonnaise,
40

Turbo Chicken Omelet, 193

Turkey:

Burger Pizza, 114

Pizza-Style Burger, 120

Roast Breast for Slicing,
92–93

Super-Balanced Baked
Omelet, 198

Vacation tips, 73

Vegetables:

Butternut Squash Soup, 27

Champion Plate, 218

Five, Salad of, 46

Ginger-Tofu Stir-Fry, 105

Lean and Mean Plate, 217

The Pump Chicken Soup,
24–25

Quinoa with, 100

Roasted, Boneless Leg of
Lamb with, 83

The Rock Plate, 223

Steamed Green and White, 124

-Tofu Soup, 26

Vegetable sides, 123–39

Baked Zucchini, 127

Brown Rice with Peas and

Carrots, 136

Crispy Sliced Potatoes, 132

Dill-and-Chive Snow Peas and
Carrots, 126

Eggplant Carpaccio, 133

Roasted Cinnamon Squash,
125

Sautéed Sliced Mushrooms
with Sun-Dried Tomatoes,
137

Sautéed Sugar Snap Peas with
Mushrooms, 130

Simply Cooked Sweet
Potatoes, 135

Spinach with Feta Cheese,
134

Steamed Green and White
Vegetables, 124

Tomato Stacks, 129

Warm Asparagus and Snow
Pea Salad, 128

Vegetarian main courses,
96–105

Asian Peanut Stir-Fry, 104

Baked Tofu, 98

Chickpea Stew with Basil, 101

Chili, 99

Ginger-Tofu Stir-Fry, 105

Kidney Bean and Butternut
Squash Stew, 102

Quinoa with Vegetables, 100

Vegetarian Special Sandwich, 35

Vinaigrettes:

Honey-Mustard Dressing, 172

Mustard-Thyme, 173

Oil and Vinegar Dressing with
Herbs, 171

Thyme, 39

Warm Asparagus and Snow Pea
Salad, 128

Watercress and Cucumber
Salad, 48

Whole Wheat Tomato Pizza, 111

Winning Quarter, 6–7

Yogurt:

Blueberries and Strawberries
with, 211

Frozen, with Protein, 212

Stewed Fruit with Orange
Juice and, 179

Yogurt Cucumber Dressing, 170

Zucchini:

Baked, 127

Hot Strips with Shallots, 207

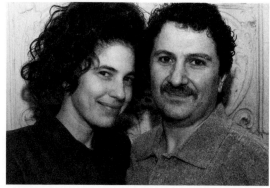

Steve and Elena Kapelonis opened their first Pump Energy Food in 1996 in New York City. Due to Pump's tremendous popularity and following, they have opened three more locations, with a fifth on the way. With over twenty-five years of culinary experience, this dynamic Greek and Jewish married couple combined their passion for healthy lifestyles and their love of delicious food to create meals that make people feel great. Acclaimed for their high-profile celebrity and fitness guru clientele, Steve and Elena are changing the way people look and feel forever. Steve and Elena live in New York City with their two daughters.